MW01294989

LETTERS OF EDWARD JENNER

The Henry E. Sigerist Supplements to the
Bulletin of the History of Medicine

New Series, no. 8
Editor: Lloyd G. Stevenson

Henry E. Sigerist, recruited by William H. Welch to be director of the Johns Hopkins Institute of the History of Medicine, was the founder of the *Bulletin of the History of Medicine* and also of the first series of supplements, which extended from 1943 to 1951. It was Sigerist's resolve that the *Bulletin* should provide the organ not only of the Johns Hopkins Institute but also of the American Association for the History of Medicine, and to this day it subserves both functions. It is therefore eminently suitable that the new series should bear the founder's name and perpetuate his scholarly interests. These interests were so broad and so varied that the supplements will recognize no narrow limits in range of theme and will publish historical essays of greater scope than the *Bulletin* itself can accommodate. It is not too much to hope that in time the Sigerist supplements will help to extend the purview of medical history.

Other Books in the New Series

1. *Almost Persuaded: American Physicians and Compulsory Health Insurance, 1912–1920,* by Ronald L. Numbers
2. *William Harvey and His Age: The Professional and Social Context of the Discovery of the Circulation,* edited by Jerome J. Bylebyl
3. *The Clinical Training of Doctors: An Essay of 1793* by Philippe Pinel, edited and translated, with an introductory essay, by Dora B. Weiner
4. *Times, Places, and Persons: Aspects of the History of Epidemiology,* edited by Abraham Lilienfeld
5. *When the Twain Meet: The Rise of Western Medicine in Japan,* by John Z. Bowers
6. *A Celebration of Medical History: The Fiftieth Anniversary of the Johns Hopkins Institute of the History of Medicine and the Welch Medical Library,* edited by Lloyd G. Stevenson
7. *Teaching the History of Medicine at a Medical Center,* edited by Jerome J. Bylebyl

An 1809 Massachusetts Vaccination Testimonial
(See Letter A-11)

LETTERS OF EDWARD JENNER

AND OTHER DOCUMENTS CONCERNING THE EARLY HISTORY OF VACCINATION

From the
Henry Barton Jacobs Collection
in the
William H. Welch Medical Library

Edited, with a Commentary and Notes, by

GENEVIEVE MILLER

Foreword by
WILLIAM R. LeFANU

THE JOHNS HOPKINS UNIVERSITY PRESS
Baltimore and London

©1983 by The Johns Hopkins University Press
All rights reserved
Printed in the United States of America

The Johns Hopkins University Press, Baltimore, Maryland 21218
The Johns Hopkins Press Ltd., London

Library of Congress Cataloging in Publication Data

Jenner, Edward, 1749–1823.
    Letters of Edward Jenner, and other documents concerning the early history of vaccination.

    (The Henry E. Sigerist supplements to the Bulletin of the history of medicine; new ser., no. 8)
    Includes index.
    1. Smallpox — Preventive inoculation — History — Sources.   2. Vaccination — History — Sources.   3. Physicians — England — Correspondence.   4. Jenner, Edward, 1749–1823. I. Miller, Genevieve.   II. Title.   III. Series.   [DNLM: W1 HE896 no. 8 / WZ 290 J54L]
R489.J5A4   1983   614.5'21   82-21295
ISBN 0-8018-2962-3

Dedicated to the memory of

HENRY E. SIGERIST

who initiated this project

CONTENTS

Letters of Edward Jenner

1785

1787

1797

1798

1799

1807

1808

1809

Appendix: Other Documents Concerning the Early History of Vaccination

FOREWORD

Fifty years ago the distinguished Baltimore physician Henry Barton Jacobs wrote about Edward Jenner: "We never get so close to a man or a woman as when we are touching and reading a letter or a note which they themselves have breathed upon and penned with their own hands. . . . Look at Jenner's carefully written pages to realize . . . what a noble, kindly, generous man he was, . . . so modest and benevolent with but the single thought in mind of wiping out of the world the greatest of all human plagues."[1] Smallpox has been eradicated at last through the campaigns of the World Health Organization, and Jenner's fame, which had suffered from excessive eulogy and unfounded invective, has finally been vindicated. Dr. Jacobs's admiration for Jenner was based on intimate familiarity; in a long career devoted to medicine and its history he had gathered a superb collection of Jennerian books and relics, including more than a hundred autograph letters, which even then were worth their weight in gold. Though Jenner described himself as "vaccination clerk to the world," only some six hundred surviving letters have been recorded and far fewer have been published — a small number when compared with the printed correspondence of other famous men, but what a large segment of the total Dr. Jacobs amassed!

All this and the rest of his rich library Dr. Jacobs generously gave in 1932 to the newly founded William H. Welch Library at the Johns Hopkins Medical Institutions. There these fascinating letters have awaited a worthy editor, though some extracts were printed by Jacobs himself and more by Dr. Genevieve Miller many years ago. Now Dr. Miller has returned to the Jenner letters and concluded a labor of love for which she is particularly fitted by profound knowledge of the history of smallpox and its prevention; she has given us a thorough scholarly edition of these important letters and their related documents. Her introduction summarizes their range and varied interest and prepares us for a feast of new and delightful information on many facets of Jenner's long career.

While Dr. Jacobs was right in recalling Jenner's virtues and his "single thought" for vaccination, the letters give evidence of his outstanding ability and his winning charm; he expressed his opinions firmly and clearly, but did not conceal his private thoughts, whether in convivial or despondent mood. Seeking, under John Hunter's guidance, the secrets of hibernation or migration and other natural history problems, he aimed, like his master, to apply the results of such research to medical advance. His colleague C. H. Parry, no mean medical scientist himself, wrote that Jenner was "capable of discerning at one glance the most obscure analogies, or of deducing the unknown and important truth from a few of the simplest but hitherto unarranged phenomena." Even beyond this Jenner had rare marks of genius: intuition, by which he "knew the answers" to his problems long before he could prove them, and readiness to adjust his conclusions in the light of new evidence, while holding firmly to his central convictions. The ablest of his contemporaries — John Hunter, Joseph Banks, Matthew Baillie, Humphry Davy — loved and admired him, respecting his intellectual and practical gifts, while the list of those who told that their work had been inspired by his includes such famous medical innovators as Laennec, Pasteur, Lister, and Pirquet. Leaders in new disciplines have claimed him as their progenitor, who cleared the way for virology, immunology, and even the whole field of preventive medicine. In reading these letters we can look over the shoulder of this friendly man, modest indeed but vastly influential, while he thinks and writes.

WILLIAM LeFANU

1. "Dedication of the Henry Barton Jacobs Room," *Bulletin of the Johns Hopkins Hospital* 50 (1932): 314–15.

INTRODUCTION

Never aim, my friend, at being a public
character, if you love domestic peace. But I
will not repine. — Nay I do not repine, but
cheerfully submit, as I look upon myself as
the instrument in the hands of that power
which never errs, of doing incalculable good
to my fellow creatures.

E. Jenner to the Rev. John Clinch,
Trinity, Newfoundland, 16 August 1805

Edward Jenner (1749–1823), the initiator and first promoter of vaccination against smallpox, was perhaps the first physician in history to receive
international acclaim during his lifetime for a new, effective medical procedure. Although great teachers like Hermann Boerhaave were known in
medical circles throughout the world, they had not conquered a single
disease; Jenner, in finding a harmless way to combat one of the world's
most dreaded diseases, had made, as John Coakley Lettsom stated, "a
Discovery of which the Records of history afford no adequate comparison,"[1]
and in addition, he had assumed the burden of instructing and urging
others to begin the practice. He became a hero to his contemporaries and
has filled a highly regarded place in medical history ever since.

Such a person inevitably becomes of intense interest to physicians and
historians alike, and every single scrap of information about him is preserved and treasured. In 1951 W. R. LeFanu published his invaluable *Bio-
Bibliography of Edward Jenner,*[2] which discusses all publications by Jenner
and lists all known letters by or to him in either manuscript or printed form.
Not available to LeFanu in a complete list, although a few had been
published and were recorded by him, were 102 Jenner letters collected by a

Baltimore physician, Henry Barton Jacobs, and presented by him to the William H. Welch Medical Library of the Johns Hopkins University in 1932.[3] Together with Harvey Cushing, a disciple and next-door neighbor of William Osler in Baltimore, Jacobs had become infected by medical history, and over the years he had built up an extensive collection of books, autograph letters, prints, and medals which embraced the history of tuberculosis, smallpox, and bacteriology. After the opening of the new Welch Medical Library in 1929, Jacobs furnished a special room with handsome mahogany cases and stained-glass windows in the third-floor Institute of the History of Medicine to house his treasures.

In addition to the 102 documents by Jenner printed here, the collection contains five letters written to him by John Hunter, which have been published elsewhere;[4] twenty-two letters from Jean de Carro to Alexander Marcet, published in 1950 by Henry E. Sigerist;[5] and letters by other contemporaries discussing vaccination. This last group of letters is published here, in the Appendix. Both the Jenner letters and the letters in the Appendix have been arranged in chronological order.

The Jenner letters are miscellaneous in character and are addressed to forty-five different correspondents. They range from the year 1785 to a few months before his death in January 1823, giving an intimate glimpse of Jenner as professional man, father, friend, country gentleman, and farmer. This correspondence permits us to look over the worried father's shoulder as he chides his son for not writing more specific information about his illness, or apologizes endlessly for long-delayed replies to medical correspondents. With letters coming in from all over the world, with little or no clerical help, he literally bore the communication burden of vaccination for a third of his life. Writing in 1804 he apologized, "It is a grievous thing to see before me Pile upon Pile of Letters unanswer'd. I really think that every hour between Sun rising & Sun-setting brings me a Letter. The pressure on my mind arising from this circumstance is painful beyond description" (Letter 15). Today we are enriched by these documents which allow us to share vicariously the thoughts and experiences of a medical country gentleman in rural Gloucestershire and Regency London.

As one would expect, the greater number of the letters relate to vaccination or its promotion, since it was this activity which brought Jenner fame and made his letters collectible. But there are also others to intimate friends or their children, to his son and nephews who assisted in business affairs, and to his patients who had written for advice. There are interesting glimpses of the customs of the time, such as entertaining colleagues at breakfast in London (Letters 68, 69, 73, 74) and exchanging gifts of herring from the shore or pheasants and gooseberries from the country (Letters 51,

99). Jenner the horticulturalist as well as the geologist is revealed in his request for apple cuttings and local rocks (Letters 52, 67, 82). As a naturalist, he received a lizard from one of his young friends (Letter 89) and carried out experiments to ascertain the value of human blood as manure for growing vegetation (Letter 2).

Among the items related to vaccination is an undated note to his close friend Thomas Pruen which gives detailed instructions on how to carry out a vaccination (Letter 102). Pruen was neither physician nor surgeon. Similarly two letters to women inoculators (Letters 16, 29) show how common it was, at least in the early days of vaccination, for laymen to perform this operation and how Jenner encouraged it.

His letters to professionals are evenly divided between physicians and surgeons. The twenty-two letters to Alexander J. G. Marcet, an Edinburgh graduate from Geneva who had settled in London, reveal Jenner sharing his thoughts with a medical colleague who not only asked professional questions about the new medical procedure, but who also served as a liaison between Jenner and physicians on the European continent. Marcet helped to bolster Jenner's two Parliamentary requests for compensation in 1802 and 1807 by sending positive reports on the success of vaccination in Denmark and France (Letters 7, 10, 23). He introduced Jenner to foreign visitors and notified him when travelers were setting out for remote areas of the world such as Abyssinia (Letters 21, 36). He commiserated when the medical politics involved in the establishment of the new National Vaccine Institution infuriated Jenner (Letters 39, 41, 42). Jenner voiced astonishment to Marcet when he received news of the de Balmis expedition sent out by the Spanish king to the New World (Letter 23). During the war with France, Jenner sought Marcet's opinion about the possibility of sending letters to Berlin and Rotterdam, while Marcet solicited Jenner's aid in obtaining the release of an English prisoner of war (Letter 60). As fellow members of the Medical and Chirurgical Society they corresponded about papers in the *Medico-Chirurgical Transactions,* of which Marcet served as editor (Letters 37, 39, 41–43). Jenner enjoyed the company of Marcet's wife, Jane, a talented author of popular science books for women and children (Letters 31, 72).

Much of the correspondence with professional colleagues includes Jenner's speculations about the origin of the cowpox virus (Letters 4, 5, 7, 15) and discusses efforts to counteract the adverse publicity propagated by the enemies of vaccination. Jenner assisted others financially in this campaign, offering to pay for the republication of an 1805 tract by a Montgomeryshire surgeon (Letter 19) and paying for the publication of the 1808 pamphlet by his young friend Thomas Charles Morgan, who defended vaccination against the attacks of the archenemy, Benjamin Moseley (Letters 49, 51). In 1810, when the antivaccinists were still publishing extensively, Jenner wrote despairingly to his London supporter Charles Murray: "[Stopping the deceptive articles and pamphlets] can't be done without some powerful Engine. But who is to construct it? One would think the statement of Facts, as they now stand before the Public from every quarter of the Globe would blow away such Stuff as these abominable People produce, like Chaff, but it is not so, or the Bills of Mortality would not exhibit weekly such horrid scenes of devastation from the Smallpox. The Legislature may perhaps be stimulated at the sight of this to take the Matter up. Indeed I think they ought as the Guardians not only of the property but the Lives of the Community" (Letter 55). Jenner believed fervently that smallpox could be exterminated from the earth and urged the formation of societies for the extermination of the smallpox throughout the Empire (Letters 13, 17, 28). He sought without success to have variolation banned by law (Letter 50).

Jenner kept in close touch with the Royal Jennerian Society in London, the publications of which he was asked to approve (Letters 12, 33–35), and he was later involved in the foundation of the National Vaccine Establishment in London. His personal problems with the latter were painfully described to friends (Letters 38, 42, 44, 45, 49). Whenever new vaccination friends appeared, such as Husson in Paris (Letter 11), Edward Jones in Montgomeryshire (Letter 19), or John Thomson in Halifax (Letter 50), Jenner made grateful comments and suggestions about how to publicize their work. He was frequently asked for cowpox vaccine (Letters 4, 5, 26, 83) and cautioned vaccinators about care in the selection of the vaccine matter and its preservation (Letters 4, 7). When questioned about the correct appearance of a vaccine pustule in its various stages, he sent a colored plate which he had had specially drawn for the purpose (Letter 6).

During the spring of 1802 he was busy soliciting testimonials in support of vaccination to present to the House of Commons in order to obtain financial support for his work (Letters 9, 10); this activity was resumed in 1806 and 1807, when a second Parliamentary grant was pending (Letters 21–24, 31).

At various times Jenner used literary assistants to help with his publications. An intriguing letter to the Reverend Thomas Frognall Dibdin in February 1805 alludes to a pamphlet which he wished to publish anonymously (Letter 18). Dibdin was to edit it and see it through the press. If such a publication does exist, it was not unearthed by W. R. LeFanu in his *Bio-Bibliography* and remains a mystery. Toward the end of Jenner's life, another literary assistant, John Fosbroke, botched his last publication, which then had to be reprinted (Letters 90, 91). Two of Jenner's nephews, the Reverend George Charles Jenner (Letters 27, 98) and the Reverend Dr. William Davies (Letter 93), at various times helped with literary or business affairs, while Charles Parry, the son of his lifelong friend Caleb Hillier Parry, assisted in his final publication (Letters 90, 91).

Jenner's international fame placed him in the position of being asked for letters of recommendation by English travelers to distant lands (Letters 33, 53). Friends also asked for personal mementos of his pioneering work. To one he sent some hair from the tail of the cow[6] that had infected the dairy maid, Sarah Nelmes, "from whose hand the Matter was taken that spread Vaccination thro' the World" (Letter 67), and to another the pen with which he was writing (Letter 96).

A number of letters to medical colleagues contain speculations about or references to various ailments, such as chronic inflammation of the liver (63), acute rheumatism (17), hydatids (63, 80), the effect of mother's milk on infants (79, 80), the presumed power of the vaccine pustule in regulating brain disorders (100), and dog distemper (37). By twentieth-century standards most of his speculations seem naive and unsophisticated, as when he observed that after one drank a glass of cider the urine smelled like it, and he then continued, "There must be a short cut from the Stomach to the Bladder. . . . What if we were to fill the Stomach of a Puppy with Mercury, first tying up the Intestine, & then give it a good squeeze?" (Letter 79).

The letters give many glimpses of Jenner's life as a country gentleman living in the shadow of Berkeley Castle, where he and his friends constructed and flew a balloon soon after the pioneering flights of Montgolfier in France (Letter 1). As a medical attendant of Lord Berkeley, who was his patron in the cause of vaccination, Jenner nervously took part in the review of his heir's credentials by the House of Lords (Letter 57). Late in life, he also served as a Berkeley magistrate, or justice of the peace, an unpaid duty of the landed gentry, who assumed responsibility for enforcing the local laws and maintaining order (Letters 60, 77, 78, 97). Until his wife's death, Jenner and his family spent several months during the "season" at nearby Cheltenham, the Gloucestershire spa popularized by King George III and his family. Here Jenner became the leading physician and acquired many new friends and patients, such as the American consul to London, General William Lyman, who died at Cheltenham under Jenner's care (Letters 58, 62). Many letters allude to the virtue of the local air and water (14, 56), and Jenner also vaccinated large numbers there, particularly among the poor (Letter 7).

With his son and close friends he shared the unique experiences into which his vaccination fame had led him, experiences such as being awarded an honorary degree from Oxford (Letter 67) and being received by the Russian Czar Alexander I during the June 1814 London visit of the victorious European leaders following the signing of the Treaty of Paris (Letter 71).

A highly sensitive man, Jenner poured out his feelings about personal tragedies. Many letters express the anxiety and grief over his elder son's death from tuberculosis (38, 46, 47, 49, 51, 53) and his continuing concern about his other son's health (67, 71, 77, 78). His wife's death was a heavy blow (Letter 76), and his own health began to deteriorate soon thereafter. A letter to Marcet (95) in the year before Jenner's death contains a detailed description of the nervous symptoms relating to sounds which preceded his fatal apoplectic attack in January 1823.

The fifteen documents in the Appendix constitute the remainder of the unpublished Jacobs material relating to Jenner or to contemporaries involved with vaccination. They originated in both the Old and New World, and even from China.

A curious document relating to Jenner's death is the last letter reproduced in the Appendix, in which Jenner's close friend, the Reverend Thomas Pruen, declared to the editor of the *Gloucester Journal* that he had been requested by Jenner to be his biographer. He therefore asked friends to send him documents, pictures, and other memorabilia for use in preparing the biography (Letter A-15). Since this letter was not published or mentioned in the *Gloucester Journal,* as requested, and since John Baron announced in the *Journal* shortly thereafter that he had been selected by Jenner's family to be Jenner's biographer, it seems clear that there were manipulations to contravene Pruen, whose dilatory nature was well known.

Three letters in the Appendix are by David Ramsay of Charleston, South Carolina, discussing both variolation and vaccination (Letters A-1, A-2, A-8). He was the principal promoter of vaccination in the South, and these letters show him distributing vaccine matter to other physicians and arguing for the widespread use of the new practice.

An embossed card from the pen of Oliver Houghton in Milton, Massachusetts, testified to the successful 1809 experiment testing the validity of vaccination through subsequent variolation (Letter A-11), while the 1810 form letter of James Smith of Baltimore sought information on the sale of lottery tickets intended to subsidize the local vaccine institution (Letter A-12). Similarly, the three letters by Corvisart, Guillotin, and Pariset give a glimpse of early vaccinations in France (Letters A-9, A-10, A-13).

One of Jenner's strongest supporters in London was John Coakley Lettsom, whose desire to see Jenner adequately rewarded led him to draw up a proposal in 1802 for a Jennerian Fund, the principal of which would continue forever "as a memorial of the Discovery of Vaccine Inoculation by Dr. Jenner" (Letter A-3). Subscriptions would be solicited throughout the entire world for "this godlike Discovery, which has for its objects, The preservation of Human existence, and the general felicity of the human race." Thus was Jenner revered. Although the Jennerian Fund never materialized, this document is a poignant reminder of the gratitude his contemporaries felt.

Lettsom also took great pains to answer queries about purported failures of vaccination (Letter A-4), helping to persuade local surgeons of its efficacy. He obtained the support of influential members of Parliament, such as Sir Henry Mildmay, who consented to become an officer of the Royal Jennerian Society after the highly publicized alleged failure of vaccination at Ringwood, Hampshire, in 1807 was clarified (Letter A-6). An additional letter from the director of the Royal Jennerian Society to the secretary of the Royal College of Surgeons concerning the Ringwood fraud, perpetrated by antivaccinist John Birch, demonstrates further the intense activity which the early days of vaccination produced (Letter A-7).

A fascinating letter from Sir George Thomas Staunton in February 1806 (Letter A-5) gives us an insight into the propagation of vaccination in China through the agency of the East India Company. The company surgeon, Alexander Pearson, wrote a treatise on the method of vaccination which Staunton translated into Chinese. It was then published and distributed free of charge at company expense.

An ironic incident comes to light in a letter (A-14) from the Scottish geologist Sir James Hall to Alexander Marcet in 1822, the final year of Jenner's life. Hall discusses the recent smallpox attack of Marcet's son, who was then living in Edinburgh, probably as a student at the university from which his father had also graduated. As the young Marcet had been vaccinated "by the great Jenner himself," the attack obviously caused consternation. Hall made it his business to call on him and "had the pleasure to find him in good health and spirits, and seemingly highly delighted with having got so well out of this terrible scrape." It is unlikely that Jenner ever learned of this.

In transcribing these letters an attempt has been made to retain the original capitalization. Contractions such as *Dr* for *Dear, Ys* and *Yrs* for *Yours, shd* for *should, wd* for *would,* and *Fd* for *Friend* have been spelled out. Otherwise the original spelling has been retained. Where possible, missing letters or words have been supplied in brackets. Apostrophes have been added when needed to indicate the possessive case and contractions, and periods have been added at the end of sentences and abbreviations. While most letters were dated by the authors, some dates have been supplied from postmarks or from information given in another hand; in such cases, the dates are in brackets. The complimentary close, which in some letters takes up three or four lines, has been run into the text of the letter as a final paragraph.

Persons are identified in a note following the first letter in which they are mentioned. Where not otherwise indicated, identifications have been derived from one or both of the following: *Dictionary of National Biography,* and William Munk, *The Roll of the Royal College of Physicians of London,* 4 vols. (London, 1878).

The major part of the research was carried out in the William H. Welch Medical Library in Baltimore, the Dudley P. Allen Medical Library in Cleveland, the National Library of Medicine in Bethesda, the Waring Library of the Medical University of South Carolina in Charleston, and the Wellcome Historical Medical Library and the British Library in London. To the very helpful staffs of all I extend sincere thanks. The skillful editing of Carolyn Moser greatly improved the manuscript.

The work was supported and publication underwritten by Public Health Service Research Grant LM 03112 from the Extramural Programs of the National Library of Medicine.

EPIGRAPH: John Baron, *The Life of Edward Jenner, M.D.,* 2 vols. (London, 1838), 2: 350–51.

1. "Lettsom's Proposal for the Jennerian Fund," Appendix, Letter A-3.

2. W. R. LeFanu, *A Bio-Bibliography of Edward Jenner, 1749–1823* (London: Harvey & Blythe, 1951).

3. "Dedication of the Henry Baron Jacobs Room," *Bulletin of the Johns Hopkins Hospital* 50 (1932): 305–17.

4. John Hunter to Edward Jenner, 22 May [1775?], published in Jessie Dobson, *John Hunter* (Edinburgh and London: E. & S. Livingstone, 1969), pp. 125–26; −6 November 1777, in Drewry Ottley, *The Life of John Hunter, F.R.S.* (Philadelphia, 1839), p. 52; −8 November 1779, in Ottley, *Hunter,* p. 59 and Baron, *Life,* 1:56; −[1785?], in Ottley, *Hunter,* p. 70, and Baron, *Life,* 1:64; −26 January, in Ottley, *Hunter,* p. 68.

5. Henry E. Sigerist, ed., *Letters of Jean de Carro to Alexandre Marcet, 1794–1817,* (Baltimore: Johns Hopkins Press, 1950), Supplements to the *Bulletin of the History of Medicine,* no. 12.

6. The Henry Barton Jacobs Collection contains a sample of the hair from this cow's tail.

SHORT TITLES

Baron, *Life* John Baron, *The Life of Edward Jenner, M.D.,* 2 vols. (London, 1838).

de Carro–Marcet
Letters Henry E. Sigerist, ed., *Letters of Jean de Carro to Alexandre Marcet, 1794–1817* (Baltimore: Johns Hopkins Press, 1950),, Supplements to the *Bulletin of the History of Medicine,* no. 12.

DNB *Dictionary of National Biography*

Fisk, *Dr. Jenner* Dorothy Fisk, *Dr. Jenner of Berkeley* (London: Heinemann, 1959).

Gent. Mag. *Gentleman's Magazine*

Jacobs, "Edward
Jenner" Henry Barton Jacobs, "Edward Jenner, a student of medicine, as illustrated in his letters," in *Contributions to Medical and Biological Research Dedicated to Sir William Osler in Honour of His Seventieth Birthday* (New York: Paul B. Hoeber, 1919), 2: 740–55.

LeFanu W. R. LeFanu, *A Bio-Bibliography of Edward Jenner, 1749–1823* (London: Harvey & Blythe, 1951). A citation such as "LeFanu 43" refers to the numbered items in the *Bio-Bibliography;* otherwise the page number is indicated.

Miller, "Letters" Genevieve Miller, "Letters of Edward Jenner," *Medical Arts and Sciences* 2 (1948): 5–17.

Munk, *Roll* William Munk, *The Roll of the Royal College of Physicians of London,* 4 vols. (London, 1878).

LETTERS OF EDWARD JENNER

1. To Dr. Caleb Hillier Parry, Bath, [ca. 1785]

My dear Friend [1]

I am sorry you can't come among us; neither Peers nor Plebeians I see can shake your Virtue.

Your directions respecting the Balloon are so clear & explicit, tis impossible for me to blunder; but to make it quite a certainty, I intend first to fill it & see if it will float in the Castle-Hall, before the publick exhibition. [2] Should it prove unwilling to mount & turn shy before a large Assembly, don't you think I may make my escape under cover of three or four dozen Squib [3] & Crackers?

I thank you for your kind offer of the Tubes & I will send a Man Thursday next to the Crosslands to fetch them. The Mouth of the Balloon is sadly torn; every other part appears sound.

Please to send me by return of Mr. Marklove [4] half a yard of such Silk as you may think most fit for the purpose. I have got some oil ready.

Pray present my respectful Comps. to Mrs. Parry, & thank her for her very friendly & polite invitation to Bath — I shall certainly come as soon as I possibly can.

Believe me Dear Doctor   ever Yours

EJ.

PS. You shall have the *Case* in full one of these days.

I shall certainly let you know the day the Balloon is to go off. Perhaps your Patients may suffer you leave them for a day. — Remember the Peer looks a little yellow sometime.

Comps. to Mr. Marklove, if you please.

1. Caleb Hillier Parry, M.D., F.R.S. (1755–1822), to whom Jenner later dedicated his *Inquiry into the Causes and Effects of the Variolae Vaccinae* (London, 1798). They were lifelong friends, having met as fellow students of the Reverend Dr. Washbourn at Cirencester. Having obtained his M.D. degree at Edinburgh in 1778, Parry entered into practice at Bath the following year and remained there throughout his life. A highly cultured man of broad

interests, he published several books on medicine and agriculture. — *DNB;* William Macmichael, *Lives of British Physicians* (London, 1830), pp. 275–304.

2. This balloon episode is discussed in Baron, *Life,* 1:69–72. It took place in Berkeley Castle.

3. *Squib:* "A paper tube or ball filled with gunpowder to be fired so as to burn and often to explode with a crack; hence, a broken firecracker the powder in which burns with a fizz." — *Webster's Collegiate Dictionary,* 1926 ed.

4. The *Post-Office Annual Directory for 1813* (London, 1813), p. 356, mentions "Marklove & Co., Berkeley Banker." It was probably his eighteen-month-old son John Marklove whose vaccination on 12 April 1798 is recorded in Jenner's *Inquiry,* p. 40.

2. To Sir Joseph Banks, 5 June 1787

Sir [1]

When I had the honor of waiting on you in London in the Spring, I promised to send you an Account of the Dog & Fox; but the Gentleman from whom I receiv'd it, not sending it so soon as I expected, occasion'd this long delay. His Account is as follows

> "I could not before this day get such intelligence as could be relyed on respecting the Dog-Fox & Terrier Bitch, which I have taken the first opportunity of transmitting to you. The Bitch did not seem very desirous of receiving the Fox at his first approaching her: But after a little amorous dalliance She came to. They copulated three times in the course of the day, and each time continued together between ten minutes & a quarter of an hour. This happen'd sometime in the month of July. It did not appear in consequence of this union that the Bitch shew'd any signs of pregnancy."

Notwithstanding this Account almost every Sportsman asserts that Foxes & Dogs will produce an Offspring. But I shall use every endeavor to set the matter clear by Experiments with these Animals. [2]

I recollect that I promis'd to send you an Account of some Experiments made on Vegitables with animal manure. I wish they were more worthy your Observation. A Person engaged in business can't conduct these matters as he would wish; his pursuits are too often interrupted. But tho' they don't go far enough to determine whether animal manure will produce lasting good effects on Vegitables, yet they prove that a superabundance of this substance is destructive to vegitable life. I shall copy the Notes as they stand on my Journal.

Feb. 10th 1780   A small quantity of the Serum of human blood was pour'd over about a square foot of grass on a grass-plot. Three sprinklings were given at the distance of a fortnight each, and the whole of the quantity applied was the Serum contain'd in forty Ounces of Blood.

April 1st   The effects it has produc'd on the vegitation of the grass is astonishing. It is beautifully green & thick & has sprung up several inches, while the surrounding grass has but just begun to shoot, & looks of a yellowish green.

May 1781   Some Mustard Seed was strew'd over thin layers of Wool in three different Tea-Saucers. The Wool in

No. 1 was moisten'd with water
No. 2 with the Serum of Blood
No. 3 with the coagulated part of the Blood mixt with Serum.

The Seeds in No. 1 sprang up soon.
In No. 2 & 3 they swell'd a little, but did not push out their Radicle — grew mouldy & died.
This Experiment was repeated with equal parts of Serum & water. A few of the Seeds just shew'd the Radicle & then died. — It was again repeated with one part Serum & two parts water. The Seeds thus treated shot & flourish'd very well.

A considerable quantity of Blood mixt with a little wood ashes & powder'd Chalk was applied round the roots of some Polyanthus Plants. The Plants soon assumed a different appearance from their neighbours. The leaves were more luxuriant & green. But about the time when the flower-stems (which were uncommonly vigorous) were push'd up to about half their usual height, they suddenly wither'd away & died.

April 21st 1782   Two young Peach Trees were manured with animal Substances. About eight pounds, or perhaps more as it was not weigh'd, were applied to the roots of each Tree. They were in a sickly state & had a very small number of Blossoms. Two Trees adjoining were very similar in appearance. The manured Trees are distinguished thus: No. 1–2   the unmanured: No. 3–4.

May 30th   From the unusual inclemency of the weather during the whole Spring, the Peach Trees in general are greatly injured & many of them appear to be destroy'd: Yet the manure above mention'd has produc'd a wonderful effect. No. 1 & 2 appear vigorous & seem to have regain'd their health, while No. 3 & 4 look sickly & have push'd out only weak & tender shoots. —

With a view of ascertaining in some measure what quantity of animal substance might be applied to a plant with woody roots to its advantage or disadvantage, the following Experiments were made:

April 20th 1782   I took four young Currant Trees of the same age, &

nearly as possible of an equal growth & appearance. They were planted in large Garden Pots of equal size in the following different substances:

No. 1 was planted in the coagulated part of fresh Blood — the surface only being cover'd with garden mould.

No. 2 was planted in equal parts of blood & common garden mould mixt together, the surface being cover'd with mould.

No. 3 was planted in common garden mould, with a Mixture of any other Substance; but this plant will from time to time be moisten'd with the Serum of blood.

No. 4 was planted in common garden mould & is to remain as a Standard without the addition of any animal substance.

The four Pots were plac'd under an east Wall, in the open Air.

April 26th   A Pint of Serum was pour'd on No. 3
May 3rd   The Serum in the same quantity applied again.
June 6th   No. 1 dead
              No. 2 nearly so
              No. 3 sickly — tho' vegitating in a small degree
              No. 4 healthy
July 20th   No. 3 recover'd — shoots & looks in full health.

By a letter from Mr. Blagden[3] I have the pleasure of being inform'd my Observations on the Cuckoo are order'd for Publication in the Phil: Trans:[4] I shall pursue the Subject during the Summer & hope to have the honour of presenting you with another paper in the Autumn; & also a paper on the exciting cause to emigration in Birds.[5]

I am Sir   with the greatest deference   Your most obedient & obliged humble Servant

Edward Jenner

Berkeley 5th June 1787

1. Jenner had been acquainted with Joseph Banks (1743–1820), the naturalist who accompanied Captain Cook's first voyage of discovery, since 1771. As a young student of John Hunter and on his mentor's recommendation, Jenner had been engaged in the processing of the specimens Banks brought back from the South Seas. The following year Jenner had declined an invitation to accompany Cook's second expedition as naturalist and instead returned to Berkeley to practice medicine. At this date, 1787, Banks was president of the Royal Society and an active promoter of scientific research. This letter, together with Banks's reply, dated 7 July 1787, was published in Baron, *Life,* 1:73–78.

2. After returning to Berkeley, Jenner was frequently called upon by Hunter to send specimens and observations relating to projects on which Hunter was working. On 26 April 1787 Hunter had read a paper entitled "Observations tending to show that the Wolf, Jackal, and Dog are all of the same Species" to the Royal Society. It is almost certain that this letter was an offshoot of the discussion of Hunter's paper. See LeFanu, pp. 8–9.

3. Charles Blagden, secretary of the Royal Society.

4. Published under the title "Observations on the Natural History of the Cuckoo," *Philosophical Transactions of the Royal Society* 78, pt. 2 (1788): 219–37. LeFanu, pp. 10–16, gives a detailed discussion of other printings and translations.

5. This was published posthumously in 1824 with the title "Some Observations on the Migration of Birds," *Philosophical Transactions of the Royal Society* 114, pt. 1 (1824): 11–44. See LeFanu, pp. 92–95, for details of other editions and translations.

3. To William Peter Lunell, Esq., Bristol, 8 October 1797

Cheltenham, October 8th 1797

You may pull and you may tug, my dear Friend,[1] but powerful as is your arm & benevolent as is your heart, it will be all to no purpose.

Can you model anew my Constitution? New arrange, new organize the particles which compose my frame? Could you, with the special authority of Omnipotence, do this, you would then take off those unfortunate eccentricities which so closely attach themselves to my Character. Forgive then my neglectfulness like a Philosopher.

The hour may come (I do not despair of its arrival) when my Stomach, where, wielding an absolute Sceptre, sits the grand Monarque of the Constitution,[2] may undergo some spontaneous change, which may meliorate its present condition; and then I trust you will find me a more orderly correspondent, and that William Shakespear may furnish me with a better motto than that which is now, alas, too applicable "To morrow, to morrow, & to morrow."

Many of your Friends, among the rest Miss Wells, reported your intention of renewing your visit to our Spa[3] — I fear we shall see no more of you this season. But at Berkeley, before the Catharine Pear Tree puts forth its leaves, I hope you will favor me with much of your society. Mrs. Jenner,[4] who by means of a roast beef Breakfast, dinner & supper has thrown off the languor that was hanging about her when you saw her at Berkeley, is soon going with me to London to spend a month or two — Little Catharine[5] accompanies us — Robert Fitzharding[6] stays at home to protect the Family Mansion. My address in Town — Robert Ladbroke's,[7] Esqr. Pall Mall.

Pray how is your amiable Wife? — the sensitive Plant? — poor John & all my old acquaintance? John, I hope goes on with his Steak & his Mutton Chops, abstaining from innutritious and indigestible matters and parting with intestinal debility. — And pray how are your Eyes? — My little Lecture on this subject did not sufficiently catch your attention. I know not why; for the preservation of this invaluable organ has occupied much of my Time, & perhaps the most intense of my Studies have been devoted to it. I shall take an early opportunity to send you Darwin's botanical Works[8] — Delightful! Don't accept them as a present, but as a mark of my chemical skill — the conversion of matter — a mineral into a vegetable.

You will scarcely understand my writing — I am in bed, confined by lameness, brought on by a violent blow on my leg.

Adieu! Believe me Yours very faithfully

Edw: Jenner

1. No information about William Peter Lunell has been uncovered. It appears from this and Letter 56 that Lunell sought Jenner's medical advice for himself and his friends. This letter has been published in an excerpted form in Jacobs, "Edward Jenner," 2:745, and also, with slight omissions, in Miller, "Letters," p. 10.

2. Jenner was convinced that the "stomach is the governor of the whole machine, the mind as well as the body." For details see Baron, *Life,* 2:93–94.

3. Cheltenham Spa, a fashionable watering place in Gloucestershire where Jenner took up residence in 1795 and practiced during the "season" for most of his subsequent life. A new study of Jenner's Cheltenham activities has recently appeared in Paul Saunders, *Edward Jenner, the Cheltenham Years 1795–1823: Being a Chronicle of the Vaccination Campaign* (Hanover, N.H.: University Press of New England, 1982). The mineral springs had been discovered in 1716 and became very popular after a visit by George III and the royal princesses in 1788.

4. Jenner had married Miss Catherine Kingscote on 6 March 1788.

5. Catherine Jenner, his daughter.

6. His infant second son, who was vaccinated on 12 April 1798, as recorded in Jenner's *Inquiry into the Causes and Effects of the Variolae Vaccinae* (London, 1798), pp. 40–41. See Letters 64, 71, 75, 77, 78, and 97.

7. Robert Ladbroke, M.P., banker of London, married Hannah Kingscote, the sister of Jenner's wife. — Thomas Dudley Fosbroke, *Berkeley Manuscripts: Abstracts and Extracts of Smyth's Lives of the Berkeleys, etc.* (London, 1821), table facing p. 218.

8. Erasmus Darwin (1731–1802), grandfather of Charles Darwin, published a very popular poem, "The Botanic Garden," in two parts: "The Loves of the Plants" (1789) and "The Economy of Vegetation" (1791).

4. To Mr. Edward Bevan, Surgeon, Stoke upon Trent, 17 October 1798

Cheltenham   17th October 1798

Sir[1]

I would with great pleasure send you some of the Cowpox Virus (as I much wish to see the Inquiry[2] prosecuted) were it in my power, but at present I have not an Atom, & greatly fear that during the continuance of the autumnal & winter months that none will be generated, as the Cow's Nipples are invold [involved] & defended by a thick Cuticle. When you proceed on your experiments on this subject, excuse my urging you to be cautious in the selection of your matter — Much confusion may arise from its being used when partially decomposed by putrefaction (see page 56 [of the *Inquiry*]), as in that case a disease would arise which would not give security from the contagion of smallpox. As cautious too should those be who prosecute the Inquiry, of using the matter which appears *spontaneously* on the Nipples of Cows.

Your observation respecting the disease's not appearing in your neighbourhood, if a dairy Country is certainly important & may tend perhap [*sic*] to elucidate that part of the subject which at present remains in some degree mysterious; I allude to the origin of the disease. I must beg you to have the goodness to tell me whether Men Servants, Carters & such as are employ'd among Horses, are also employ'd as Milkers of Cows.

In Scotland as well as Ireland, it seems no Men Servants are employ'd in the dairy. This tends to strengthen what I so strongly suspect that the disease arises from morbid matter generated by a Horse.[3]

When I see my Nephew, I shall certainly present your Compliments.

I am Sir   Your very obedient Servant

E. Jenner

Be kind enough to direct to me at Cheltenham.

1. Edward Bevan (1770–1860), who later distinguished himself as a scientific apiarian through his book *The Honey-Bee: its Natural History, Physiology, and Management* (1827), which went through three editions. Trained in surgery as an apprentice to a surgeon in Hereford and at St. Bartholomew's Hospital, he obtained his M.D. degree from St. Andrew's University in 1818. This letter was published in Miller, "Letters," p. 11.

2. Jenner's *Inquiry into the Causes and Effects of the Variolae Vaccinae* (London, 1798), which had been published at the end of June.

3. At this time Jenner believed that a disease called the grease, which attacked the heels of horses, and cowpox were the same. He thought that the infection was transferred to cows by men who both attended horses and worked in dairies. See Jenner, *Inquiry*, pp. 2–3, 46–49.

5.   To Jean de Carro, Vienna, 27 November 1799

Berkeley, November 27th 1799

Sir[1]

I scarcely know an occurrence since the commencement of my Inquiry into the nature of the Variolae Vaccinae that has given me greater satisfaction than the reception of your Letter.[2] It breathes the true spirit of philosophic candour, & has placed its author high in my estimation.

Conscious of its importance it was always my hope that the subject would be taken up on the Continent, and I am much gratified to see it fall into such able hands in Vienna; for I never had a fear of its failure but from its being conducted by those who were incapable of making just discriminations.

I cannot forbear congratulating you on the success you have already met with, altho it must be confess'd that congratulation bears hard upon egotism. From the state of your Patient's arm when you wrote your Letter, it seem'd clear that you would succeed in reproducing the disease with the matter you found upon the Linen, yet, having now some five Cases before me, I have enclos'd two portions of the Virus taken from different subjects; & with the view of excluding Oxygen as much as possible, I have plac'd it between two pieces of Glass. The quantity is larger than it appears, as so much evaporation takes place in drying. When you make use of it, moisten it either by taking up a very small portion of water on the point of your Lancet, or by breathing upon it.

Lest you should not have seen my second Pamphlet on the subject,[3] I have directed a friend in London to send one of them to Lord Grenville's office[4] directed for you. Should you not receive it, conclude that it is out of print. Shortly, it is my intention to republish the two Pamphlets with an Apendix & shall take a pleasure in conveying them to you the earliest opportunity that offers.[5]

If the Cowpox be unknown in the Country in which you dwell, I should presume that Men Servants, who are employ'd among Horses, are not employ'd in milking Cows. In Ireland, & in Scotland, where the Men Servants do not milk, the disease is also unknown. It is unlucky (if I am right in my opinion of the origin of the disease) that we cannot communicate it in a *direct* way from the Horse to the Cow. But even the matter of Cowpox, when taken from the Nipple of one Cow & inserted into that of another by the point of a Lancet, produces no disease; at least no effect has follow'd its application in any instance that has come to my knowledge. So that there is probably some undiscover'd agent operating to give effect to the *equine* virus.

After reading my Publication and observing my assertion that the Cowpox does not produce Pustules, you may probably ere now have been much surpris'd at finding that they appear'd in considerable abundance among the Patients, inoculated with the virus taken from a Cow, at the Smallpox Hospital in London.[6] However I presume this surprise will cease

10

when you are inform'd that on the 5th day after the Cowpox Virus had been inserted into one arm, the variolous virus was inserted into the other, in those whose eruptions resembled those of smallpox; & thus, in my opinion, the two diseases became blended. The Pustules, as the disease made its progress from one Patient to another soon began to decrease in number, and now they are become quite extinct, the matter producing appearances exactly similar to that newly taken from the Pock on the Nipple of the Cow. How extremely curious & singular is this Fact! Does it not almost tell us that the Cowpox is the original disease, the Smallpox a Variety & being the weaker is driven off by the stronger? or is the latter assimilated by the former?

Conceiving it possible that the pamper'd London Cow (from which the Virus was taken to the Smallpox Hospital) might generate it in some respects different from the Animal that ranges, more in a state of Nature, over our pastures in the Country (from which source I had been accustomed to make my Experiments) I procured some from a Cow at one of the Farms on the confines of London. But altho' this matter has been passing from one person to another for the space of several months & upwards of two hundred Persons have been inoculated from this source, yet no Pustules have appear'd among any of them. I do not mean to say that no rashes or eruptions of any sort have attended the disease. When the *Areola* has spread wide around the inoculated Pustule I have sometimes seen a rash upon the Patient, and sometimes several pimples, small, hard & of a redish colour have shewn themselves on different parts of the body, some of which have contain'd a perceptible fluid at their apex. But this appearance is very rare, and I imagine takes place on the same principal as when excited by the local stimulus of many acrid substances. For example, the local inflammation & irritation of Cantharides, Burgundy Pitch, Emetic Tartar & many other irritating substances will as often produce general affections of the skin as the virus of the Cowpox; indeed I think more often.

I should be extremely happy to furnish you with matter immediately from the Cow, but in this part of our Island I have not heard of the existence of the disease among Cattle for several months past. What I have sent I hope may retain its activity till it arrives at Vienna — My best wishes accompany it. The Glasses are dated to show you how long the matter has been taken from the arm.

I shall not trouble you with a detail of Cases, but in a word shall inform you that in this Island the numbers inoculated with vaccine virus already exceed five thousand. Nothing has occurr'd to lessen the confidence I at first held out; on the contrary fresh & convincing evidence of the powers of the vaccine disease in destroying the effects of the variolous is constantly flowing in. I hope to be favor'd with your correspondence & remain, Dear Sir, your obedient humble Servant

Edw: Jenner

1. Jean de Carro (1770–1857) from Geneva had obtained his M.D. degree from Edinburgh in 1793. Intending originally to practice in his home city, he went instead to Vienna because of the political upheaval in Geneva caused by the French Revolution. He was influential in introducing vaccination to continental Europe, the Near East, and India. See *de Carro–Marcet Letters.* Part of this letter was published in Miller, "Letters," p. 12.

2. De Carro's letter of 14 September 1799 from Vienna is published in Baron's *Life,* 1:334.

3. *Further Observations on the Variolae Vaccinae, or Cow Pox* (London: Printed by Sampson Low, 1799). (LeFanu 45.)

4. William Wyndham Grenville (1759–1834), who was secretary of state for foreign affairs at this time.

5. This was the second edition of the *Inquiry,* published in 1800 (LeFanu 21).

6. These vaccinations were performed by William Woodville, physician to the Small Pox and Inoculation Hospital in London. For an account of Woodville's experiments see his *Reports of a Series of Inoculations for the Variolae Vaccinae, or Cow-Pox; with Remarks and Observations on this Disease, Considered as a Substitute for the Small-Pox* (London: James Phillips and Son, 1799). Jenner restated his opinion that cowpox would not produce variolous pustules in his third treatise on vaccination, *A Continuation of Facts and Observations Relative to the Variolae Vaccinae, or Cow Pox* (London: Printed by Sampson Low, 1800). All of these pamphlets are reprinted in Edgar M. Crookshank, *History and Pathology of Vaccination,* 2 vols. (London, 1889), vol. 2. For a recent discussion of the possible contamination of Jenner's cowpox vaccine see Peter Razzell, *Edward Jenner's Cowpox Vaccine: The History of a Medical Myth* (Firle, Sussex: Caliban Books, 1977).

6.   To J. Barwis, Esq., Temple, [ca. 1800]

My dear Sir[1]

The Plate I have sent[2] shews the progress of the Vaccine Pustule. Long exposure to light has somewhat lessen'd the brightness of the tints surrounding them. You must look sharp for the dates, which are nearly obliterated — you will find them in the Centre between the two Columns one of which represents the Smallpox, the other the Vaccine.

If your Friend has any doubts or fears, I will inspect the arms with great pleasure.

Truly Yours

E. Jenner

N.B.   The progress of the Pustules is not always *exactly* the same.

1. Mr. Barwis has not been identified, but he was probably a surgeon. He is also mentioned in Letters 23 and 25.

2. This is probably Plate C, discussed in LeFanu, pp. 55–56.

7. To Dr. Alexander J. G. Marcet, London, 11 November 1801

Cheltenham, November 11th 1801

Dear Sir[1]

I am extremely sorry to think how much time has elapsed since you did me the favor of writing and enclosing a Letter for my perusal from Copenhagen. The great extent of my correspondence upon the Vaccine Subject, join'd with my professional engagements, frequently throws me into some confusion. I am now so far behind hand, that full forty Letters lie before me unanswer'd. Let this, Sir, in some measure plead my excuse for this long delay. The Letter you have done me the honor to lay before me certainly contains some curious information. It is highly probable that the Cowpox must have been known among Mankind for Centuries past; indeed from the time that Horses, Cows & Men associated, as in the Farms in the West of England; that is, where the Men Servants officiated in the double capacity of Carters & Milkers.[2] Where this association is not form'd, we know nothing of the Cowpox. Since my residence at Cheltenham this Summer, I have suffer'd the poor people, both in the Town and the neighbouring Villages, to come here and be inoculated. Vast numbers have approach'd me and among them I have seen several decisive illustrations of the truth of my doctrine relative to the origin of the Vaccine Disease. On the hand of a Carter who twenty years ago received the infection from the heel of a Horse, & who has now repeatedly resisted the vaccine infection, are three Cicatrices, precisely like those which appear on the Arm, after the inoculation for the Cowpox.

I should be happy to see your evidence from Copenhagen before the Public.[3] With respect to Eruptions following the Inoculation, I must remark that it is an occurrence which takes place so very rarely, when the process is properly conducted, as not to merit attention. I have reason to think that Virus taken from a Pustule in its declining state, will frequently produce anomalies; among others, the spurious Pustule. The time of taking the Virus for inoculation is one of the most important points for our attention in vaccine Inoculation. Pray impress this upon the minds of your foreign Correspondents. [*Footnote in another hand:* "From the 5th to 9th day is the time Dr. Jenner recommends."] I want to make a thousand observations to you on the subject, but as I expect so soon to return to London, I shall hope for the pleasure of seeing you in Bond Street[4] when it may be more advantageously resumed.

Be assured that I am   Dear Sir   very faithfully Yours

E. Jenner

1. Alexander J. G. Marcet (1770–1822), from Geneva, had obtained his M.D. degree at Edinburgh and entered medical practice in London. He was in close touch with many scientists on the Continent, including his fellow Genevan Jean de Carro in Vienna. See *de Carro–Marcet Letters*. Eighteen letters which Jenner wrote to Marcet are preserved in the Library of the Royal Society of Medicine in London. See also Letters, 10, 15, 21, 23, 25, 31, 32, 36, 37, 39, 41–43, 53, 60, 63, 70, 72–74, 95, and A-14.

2. The origin of the vaccinia virus is still a mystery. The most recent analysis and hypothesis is by Derrick Baxby, *Jenner's Smallpox Vaccine: The Riddle of Vaccinia Virus and Its Origin* (London: Heinemann, 1981).

3. This probably refers to the article by E. Viborg, "Experiments made for the Purpose of proving that the Small-pox is a Disease common both to Men and Brutes," *Medical and Physical Journal*, 8 (September 1802): 271–73.

4. Jenner stayed in Bond Street when he came to London.

8. To Lady Berkeley, 1 January 1802

January 1 1802
Bond St. [London]

Dear Lady Berkeley[1]

Just as I was about to make up my packet for your Ladyship, in which *was to have been* enclos'd Mr. Foley's Letter, in rush'd no less a number than thirteen Letters. No wonder then at my being for a moment confused; but you have got it now & all is well. Respecting Letters & my present *uncommon caution about them*, I shall draw up a certificate which shall be sign'd by Mrs. Jenner. — Wathen.[2] I set myself up you know for a bit of a Physiognomist. The next time you see H. Hicks[3] pray ask him what I said of this *Gentleman* the first time I ever saw him, which was at Eastington.[4] I think it was exactly this, "that the Knave, the Fool & the cunning Man were blended together, & made the disagreeable compound I then beheld. I remember the circumstance of the Church — Something like his representation certainly took place & I am glad he could discern that I had no inclination for his Society.

The Natives of the County resident in London seem disposed to join *the List*. One of them, a respectable Gentleman of the Law, call'd upon me this morning & ask'd if it would not be prudent to insert a Copy of the advertisement & the list of the Names, from the Glocester Journal of Monday last,[5] in a London Paper & at the same time mention the name of some Banker who should receive subscriptions? I could only reply that it was not in my power to give a decisive answer, but that I should immediately inquire at the place most proper to communicate intelligence on this subject. Your Ladyship will have the kindness to think of this, & let me know.

Will Lord Berkeley be good enough to write to the Archbishop of Canterbury? He is a native of the County. Should not we consider all natives of Glostershire, as proper to be applied to? — Taylor is out with a very good Paper on the merits of the Cowpox Inoculation in the Medical Journal of this day.[6] Shrapnell[7] may not now be at the Castle, I shall therefore send it to you.

After your Ladyship has perused the subjoined Certificate you will not be afraid to trust me with a sight of Wathen's Letter.

With a due sense of the obligations you place me under I remain
Your Ladyship's very humble Servant

E. Jenner

This is to certify that my Husband Dr. Jenner is become extremely careful of every Letter he receives from his Correspondents.

Witness my hand   Cath. Jenner

1. Mary Cole, daughter of William Cole of Wotton-under-Edge in Gloucestershire, had married Frederick Augustus, fifth Earl of Berkeley, on 16 May 1796. She continually supported Jenner in his fight to obtain the acceptance of vaccination. Jenner's father had been vicar of Berkeley, had tutored Frederick Augustus' father, and there was always a very close connection between the two families.

2. No positive identification. Samuel Wathen, Esq., of Woodchester, near Berkeley, was appointed sheriff of Gloucestershire for the year 1803. — *Gent. Mag.* 73, pt. 1 (1803): 185.

3. Henry Hicks was a lifelong friend of Jenner who lived in Eastington, six miles from Berkeley. He had advised Jenner to publish his *Inquiry* privately after the Royal Society took no action, and he was frequently consulted when Jenner was preparing it for publication. Hicks' two children were the first whom Jenner inoculated in November 1798, when he was again able to obtain cowpox virus. See Baron, *Life,* 1:142. Later Hicks published a pamphlet defending Jenner from the attack by Dr. George Pearson: *Observations on a late Publication of Dr. Pearson, entitled, an Examination of the Report of the Committee of the House of Commons, on the Claims of Remuneration for the Vaccine Pock Inoculation* (Stroud: W. S. Wilson, 1803).

4. In addition to Hicks, Jenner's friend Richard Worthington and his brother-in-law, the Reverend William Davies, vicar of Eastington, resided there.

5. The residents of Gloucestershire, led by the Earl of Berkeley and Jenner's close friends, drew up a testimonial of their great appreciation of his discovery. The *Glocester Journal,* 21 December 1801, states: "Many of the Noblemen and most respectful Gentlemen of the County of Glocester having expressed a wish that some public Acknowledgment should be made to Dr. JENNER, for his singularly happy and ingenious Discovery of VACCINE INOCULATION: — We, the undersigned, desirous of promoting so laudable and so patriotic a Design, have commenced a Subscription for carrying the same into Effect. . . . We trust it will only be the Prelude to a Remuneration in some Degree adequate to his Deserts, and to which he has the best-founded Claim on the Gratitude of the British Nation." In this instance the financial contributions were used to purchase a service of plate, appropriately engraved with a figure of Apollo destroying Python. See Baron, *Life,* 1:481 f., and *Public Characters of 1802–1803* (London, 1803), p. 42.

6. *The Medical and Physical Journal* (London) 7 (1802): 11–12, signed D.T., urged that Jenner be remunerated by his country for his discovery. David Taylor, surgeon of Wotton-under-Edge, Gloucestershire, testified for Jenner when his petition for remuneration was brought before Parliament. See *Report from the Committee on Dr. Jenner's Petition respecting his Discovery of Vaccine Inoculation,* (London, 1802), pp. 32–33.

7. William F. Shrapnell, surgeon to the South Gloucestershire militia, was a close friend of Jenner. See Fisk, *Dr. Jenner,* p. 110.

9.   To [Dr. James Currie, Liverpool,] 10 March 1802

Bond St. London
10th March 1802

Sir [1]

Knowing that you have long been a promoter of Vaccine Inoculation & that under your protection it has been carried to a great extent in Liverpool & its environs,[2] I take the liberty to request the favor of you to send me the general result of the practice. The Subject will (I believe in the early part of the ensuing week) undergo a Discussion before an august Assembly,[3] & I should like to be prepared with a full body of evidence from authorities the most respectable.

I have nothing new to communicate on the subject or I should do myself the pleasure of laying it before you. The enclos'd Paper of Instructions[4] I have drawn up, & distributed for the use of those who have taken up the Vaccine Lancet without knowing or considering that discretion was necessary to direct its use. Some mischief has arisen from indiscretion; but on the whole, less than I could expect, the practice having spread so rapidly & so widely & having occasionally pass'd into such bungling hands. I wish, Sir, I could congratulate you on the adoption here of the means you had the happiness a few years ago to announce, for extinguishing the flame of Typhus.[5] I have often been bold enough to say, that the timidity & supiness [*sic*] of the London Practitioners in not bringing it into use,[6] while such numbers perish daily under the common routine of practice, deserve the severest reproach: but I can make no impression.

I have the honor to be   with great respect   Sir   Your obedient humble Servant

E. Jenner

1. Although unaddressed, this letter is undoubtedly written to James Currie (1756–1805), a prominent Liverpool physician, who in addition to medical publications wrote the first biography of his fellow Scot Robert Burns.

2. For an account of the early history of vaccination in Liverpool, see Robert Willan, *On Vaccine Inoculation* (London: Richard Phillips, 1806), Appendix, pp. xiv f.

3. On 17 March 1802 Jenner presented a petition to the House of Commons to be remunerated for his discovery. He was granted £10,000 at this time, and another petition in 1807 yielded £20,000. See Baron, *Life*, 1:484–510.

4. Jenner's *Instructions for Vaccine Inoculation* (London: Printed by D. N. Shury, n.d.), a quarto sheet (LeFanu 60) which was printed between November 1801 and February 1802. See LeFanu, pp. 60–62.

5. In 1797 Currie had published his *Medical Reports on the Effects of Water, Cold and Warm, as a Remedy in Fever and febrile Diseases* (Liverpool: Cadell & Davies, 1797).

6. Currie's son commented on this phenomenon in his biography of his father: William Wallace Currie, *Memoir of the Life, Writings, and Correspondence of James Currie, M.D., F.R.S. of Liverpool*, 2 vols. (London, 1831), 1:221.

10. To Dr. Alexander J. G. Marcet, London, 22 March 1802

Bond St. Monday

My dear Sir[1]

Many thanks to you for your obliging Communication from Copenhagen.[2] It will answer a very good purpose in the Committee of the House of Commons.[3] I fear it will not be in my power to dine with you on the day you mention, as the important business which now occupies my attention will hardly be then at an end.

With much respect   Yours dear Sir   very truly

E. Jenner

1. See Letter 7, n. 1.

2. The king of Denmark had appointed a committee headed by Frederik Christian Winsloew (1752–1811) to investigate vaccine inoculation and to formulate regulations for its application. Baron (*Life*, 1:475–78) gives an abstract of the committee's report of 19 December 1801. The recommendations, which provided for free vaccination of soldiers and their families, sailors, students in public schools, and the poor, were accepted by the king, who commanded that they be enforced.

3. See Letter 9, n. 3.

11. To − − −, Paris, 10 April 1802

Sir[1]

I take this opportunity of sending you a line by my Friend Dr. Marshall,[2] to express to you the high obligations you have placed me under by the many handsome allusions you have made to my name in your late Publication on Vaccine Inoculation.[3] Your Work, Sir, on this interesting subject is not only elegant, but it must necessarily prove of great public utility. It is one of those mass Clubs which I wish to see powerful arms, like yours, take up in all Countries to crush the horrid Monster Smallpox. I have the happiness to tell you that the pretty general introduction of the Vaccine in our Metropolis has already manifestly diminish'd the number of Victims to the Casual Smallpox. I trust the Metropolis of France can boast of a similar gratification.

I have the honor to be, Sir   Your obedient & obliged humble Servant
Edwd. Jenner

London 10th April 1802

1. This letter was probably addressed to Henri-Marie Husson (1772–1853), who had personal communication with Jenner in February 1802, but see n. 3 below. See LeFanu, pp. 112, 147. See also Letters 66 and A-9.

2. Dr. Joseph H. Marshall from Eastington, was a friend of Henry Hicks, had practiced at Stonehouse, near Berkeley, and was one of the first to learn how to vaccinate from Jenner. In July 1800 upon the recommendation of Dr. John Walker, who assisted him, Marshall began vaccinating the crew of the Royal Naval ship *Endymion*. Between then and January 1802 he toured the Mediterranean and carried out vaccinations at Gibraltar, Minorca, Malta, Sicily, Naples (where he became physician extraordinary to the king of Naples), Rome, Leghorn, and Genoa. Marshall was journeying to Paris to take up residence there. See "Medical and Physical Intelligence," *Medical and Physical Journal* 7 (May 1802): 480, "Continuation of the Evidence delivered before the Committee of the House of Commons, in Support of Dr. Jenner's Application for Parliamentary Reward," ibid. 8 (1802): 22–24; Baron, *Life*, 1:395–403; John Epps, *The Life of John Walker, M.D.* (London, 1832), pp. 36–72.

3. Probably H. M. Husson, *Recherches historiques et médicales sur la vaccine* (Paris, an IX [1801]); but another possible addressee of this letter was François Colon, who in 1801 published *Essai sur l'inoculation de la vaccine* (Paris, an IX).

12.   To [John Addington, London, ca. 1803]

My dear Sir[1]

Your first Comparative Statement,[2] your second, and everything you have exhibited on that subject, has been mark'd with clearness & precision sufficient for any *common* Head to comprehend; but my opinion is that it should be thrown into that form which will best suit the *uncommon* Head, the uncommonly dull. Arranged with Chevy Chase, & the Babes in the Wood[3] on Cottage Walls, it should assume the simplest Form possible in order to be intelligible to those who will seek its perusal there. The enlighten'd, it is to be hoped, have already (from thinking of Vaccination) beheld its comparative advantages. All this consider'd, I am inclin'd to think that, after they have received some of your finishing touches, the perpendicular Columns will be the best.[4] I don't mean to suggest that it should assume the shabby, cropt form, in which it now lies before me — I should vote it on a handsome Quarto. It is beneath the Society to think on pence.[5]

Allow me to congratulate you & all lovers of the Vaccine, on the introduction of our little *Pearl* into India.[6] This intelligence reach'd me yesterday from De Carro at Vienna[7] & from a Gentleman just arrived from Madras.
[Remainder of page missing.]

1. Although the addressee's name does not appear on the letter, it is unquestionably written to John Addington, surgeon, who resided at Spital Square, London. In 1801 he had published *Practical observations on the inoculation of the cow-pox: to which is prefixed a compendious history of that disease, and of its introduction as a preventive of the small-pox* (Birmingham: J. Belcher, 1801).

2. J. Addington, *A comparative view of the natural small-pox, inoculated small-pox, and inoculated cow-pox, in their effects on individuals and society,* published by order of the Medical Council of the Royal Jennerian Society ([London]: Nichols, [1803]). This was also published in a smaller format with minor changes ca. 1804, published in German in Vienna ca. 1804, and published in a Portuguese edition of the second edition of Jenner's *Inquiry* in Lisbon in 1803. In 1810 it was reprinted in Charles Maclean, *On the state of vaccination in 1810* (London, 1810), pp. 104–5, with the comment: "If the statements I have made be correct, not only is this comparative view, published by order of the Jennerian Society, in all its material parts, erroneous, but, in many, the very reverse of truth" (pp. 105–6).

3. "Chevy Chase" and "Babes in the Wood" were popular ballads which first appeared in printed form in the eighteenth century.

4. The publication was arranged in tabular form.

5. The Royal Jennerian Society was founded on 19 January 1803 as a charitable organization to carry out free vaccination of the poor. Under the patronage of royalty and heavily endowed by voluntary contributions it supported a house in Salisbury Square where John Walker was the resident inoculator. The *Gentleman's Magazine* reported its "Festival" on 17 May 1803, when "300 noblemen & gentlemen assembled at the Crown & Anchor Tavern." — *Gent. Mag.* 73, pt. 1 (1803): 461–66.

6. According to Baron (*Life,* 1:420) vaccine matter reached India on 31 March 1802.

7. See Letter 5.

13.   To T. Cobb, Esq., Banbury, Oxfordshire, 8 March 1803

Hertford St. May Fair[1]
March 8th 1803

My dear Sir[2]

I rec'd your first obliging Letter at Berkeley just upon my setting off for London & put it by so *very carefully* among some of my Packages that it has as yet resisted my endeavors to bring it forth; however it is safe *somewhere,* & I shall pay your benevolent Contribution into the general Fund of the R. J.

Institution for the extermination of the Smallpox.[3] The example you have so handsomely set to People in the Country, I hope will be follow'd by others, and let me tell you for your honor & Credit that you lead the way as a Subscriber out of the Metropolis — But my opinion is, that the Metropolis is the very Focus of Infection, & that destroying the Disease here will be essential in lessening its calamaties in the Country. We hope soon to see Societies form'd throughout the Empire for the Extermination of the Smallpox, cooperating with that which we hope soon to see in full & effective action here.

Accept my warmest acknowledgements for your kind congratulations. Honours certainly fall in showers upon me, but Emoluments fall off. You who possess a generous heart will feel indignant when I tell you that those identical People who last year brought their Children to me to be inoculated, now take their new born Little ones to their domestic Surgeon or Apothecary for that purpose — and why? They save perhaps a few Guineas by the exchange.

However I trust you know me too well to suppose that I feel a moment's disquietude at events like these. They clearly shew the fallacy of Mr. Addington's[4] prediction, who express'd a confidence in my soon remunerating myself by the numbers who would flock to me for Inoculation.

Mrs. Jenner begs her best Comps. & I remain   with best wishes Yours very faithfully

E. Jenner

1. Jenner had just taken a house in London and entered into practice there. The enterprise did not bring the financial reward he had anticipated, and he soon returned to the country. See Baron, *Life*, 2:3-4. The second paragraph of this letter was published in Miller, "Letters," p. 13.

2. T. Cobb and his wife were patients of Jenner whom he had probably met at Cheltenham. See Letters 47 and 48.

The Jacobs collection possesses the following prescription written by Jenner in January 1800:

"Mr. Cobb will probably find advantage from the use of Rhubarb join'd with a little James's powder — for example — He may take two grains of James's powder & five of Rhubarb every night & if this should not be felt sensibly by the Bowels four or five grains of Rhubarb may be taken daily about noon.

"NB. Small Blisters perpetuel

"Dr. Jenner at Mr. Paytherus's, Adam Street, Adelphi, London."

3. See Letter 12, n. 5.

4. Henry Addington (1757-1844), at this time prime minister and chancellor of the Exchequer, who had urged that Jenner be awarded no more than £10,000, since the public honor granted by Parliament constituted "a reward that would last forever, and also that the comfort of his family would be amply provided for in his extended practice." See G. C. Jenner, *The Evidence at Large, as laid before the Committee of the House of Commons, respecting Dr. Jenner's Discovery of Vaccine Inoculation* (London, 1805), pp. 194-95.

14.   To Dr. Caleb Hillier Parry, Physician, Circus, Bath, 17 August 1804

My dear Doctor[1]

You are entitled to the thanks of the luckless Co for your exertions.

I lose not a Post in complying with your request & hope the business will be got thro' with all convenient speed.

It is to be fear'd that the Norfolk St. Commodity is not marketable — Where is it to be found?

This place is uncommonly crowded[2] — The more I see of C. Fox,[3] the more I admire him. I had no notion that, *off the Stage*, he possess'd such a playful Mind.

Yours truly

EJ.

Cheltenham 17 August 1804

1. See Letters 1, 17, and 57.
2. The Jenners went regularly to Cheltenham for three or four months during the "season," and Jenner was actively in practice there. A friend described his various residences: "It is worthy of record, that the house which he inhabited on his first settling in Cheltenham, is situated opposite a drug shop, in the lower part of the High Street, then considered a capital but now an inferior residence; afterwards he resided at No. 8, in St. George's Place. For some years he was the sole physician of note in the town, being used to spend some part of the year in it, and the remainder at Berkeley." — John Fosbroke, "Local Biography," in T. D. Fosbroke, *A Picturesque and Topographical Account of Cheltenham, and its Vicinity* (Cheltenham, 1826), pp. 295–96. See Paul Saunders, *Edward Jenner: The Cheltenham Years, 1795–1823* (Hanover, N.H.: University Press of New England, 1982).
3. Charles James Fox (1749–1806), a prominent statesman famous for his oratorical skills, who became a friend of Jenner. — Baron, *Life*, 2:305. For details see Saunders, *Edward Jenner*.

15.   To Alexander J. G. Marcet, 3 September 1804

My dear Sir[1]

I am sorry to be under the necessity of acknowledging that there are great numbers of Gentlemen who have reason to complain of my tardiness as a Correspondent; but you see, I am determin'd that you shall not make one of this long & tremendous list. It is a grievous thing to see before me Pile upon Pile of Letters unanswer'd. I really think that every hour between Sun rising & Sun-setting brings me a Letter. The pressure on my mind arising from this circumstance is painful beyond description. You will say it is a singular Fact, but I do assure you our Friend De Carro[2] has increased these painful sensations in no inconsiderable degree by his great attention to me. Be assured he shall be among the first (for his civilities & his labors in the Vaccine Cause entitle him to preeminence) to whom I shall address a *long* Letter. Should you chance to write to him before me, pray tell him this — but I don't despair of sending him a line by the conveyance you mention.

Allow me to thank you for your very friendly Letter. I certainly never should have asserted in terms so positive the Fact relative to the origin of the *Vaccine* Matter, had I not satisfied myself that I was correct. There was a circumstance in my first Publication which escaped the attention of almost all my Readers, perhaps even you, and that is my second Plate;[3] which represents a Pustule on the arm from virus derived from the *Horse* & not the *Cow*. — The Paper I inserted in the Med: & Ph: Journal for August[4] I hope will attract attention. Since writing it, a Case has come to my knowledge of smallpox by *contagion*, after the inoculation of the disease, which inoculation had occasion'd what is call'd a *bad* arm, & affected the System considerably. I have at this time under my Eye a Child with the Tinea Capitis[5] who has [on] one arm an imperfect Pustule, & on the other, one that is in every respect complete. — With Comps. to Mrs. Marcet.[6]

Yours dear Sir   very faithfully

E. Jenner

Cheltenham, 3 Sept. 1804

1. See Letter 7, n. 1.
2. See Letter 5.
3. This faces p. 36 in the first edition of Jenner's *Inquiry* (1798).
4. *Medical and Physical Journal* 12 (August 1804): 97–102. Jenner reprinted this article two years later: *On the Varieties and Modifications of the Vaccine Pustule, Occasioned by an Herpetic State of the Skin* (Cheltenham: H. Ruff, 1806). (LeFanu 79–81.)
5. Ringworm of the scalp.
6. Jane Marcet (1769–1858), the daughter of a wealthy Swiss merchant living in London, had married Alexander Marcet on 4 December 1799. She wrote popular books on science and political economy for the general public and children.

16.   To [Mrs. David Pennant], Downing near Holywell, Flintshire, 30 September [1804?]

Cheltenham 30th September

Dear Madam[1]

I am happy to find that you have taken up the vaccine inoculation & hope you will go on as successfully with it as your Sister in Hampshire. The

Case you mention to me of your first patient somewhat puzzles me as I do not recollect ever meeting with one similar to it. But I conceive that the Child is of a very irritable habit and that even the little irritation excited by the Pustule on the arm so early as the 10th day produc'd the blotches you describe which so quickly vanish'd, & which I presume might be call'd the Nettle Rash. This irritation, I imagine, has never subsided from its commencement & has occasion'd that variety of Symptoms you describe.

The method you have taken will probably subdue it. On any similar occasion, or whenever the arm is much disposed to inflame, I would recommend your checking its progress by applying something to act upon the Pustule. Goulard's Extract in its undiluted state will answer your purpose very well. Into a Vial of it you may dip a Probe or a Skewer & thus apply it upon the Pustule, or you may apply a single Drop upon it at once & suffer it to remain on two or three minutes. This may be repeated two or three times a day and if the Extract be good it will so alter the nature of the Pustule that you will not be annoy'd with inflammation or its consequences. In case of itching when very troublesome, a Rag dipp'd in Vinegar & Water makes a good application. When the Scab comes off prematurely & leaves a sore, let it be touch'd now & then with the Goulard Extract which will soon renew it.

Pray have the kindness to write again soon, that I may know how this Case has terminated. — You will find the matter most active in the early stages of the Pustule — for example, on the 6th, 7th, and 8th days. — Does Dr. Currie[2] know this? — It would have afforded me great pleasure had I seen you in London. I shall be more fortunate I hope on another occasion. Lady P[eyton][3] left us a few days ago; better I hope for the Cheltenham Water.

Pray remember me to Mr. Pennant & Miss Charlotte and believe me dear Madam

Your very faithful humble Servant

E Jenner

I am particularly desirous of seeing the C.P.[4] properly managed at Chester,[5] as I have heard that Small pox Matter was once sent there by mistake for the C. Pox.

1. All the personal names except that of Dr. Currie have been scratched out in this letter, but it is possible to reconstruct them. From the address, Jenner's correspondent is undoubtedly the daughter-in-law of Thomas Pennant, the well-known Welsh naturalist and traveler who had died in 1798, and whose son David (d. 1841) succeeded his father at Downing and edited his posthumous publications. In 1808 Jenner sent her a copy of his *Facts . . . respecting Variolous Contagion.* — LeFanu, p. 74.

2. See Letter 9. Since Currie died on 31 August 1805, this letter was probably written in 1803 or 1804.

3. Lady Frances Peyton was the sister of Sir John Rous, M.P., who was brother-in-law to Thomas Kingscote, the brother of Jenner's wife. She was an early supporter and practitioner of vaccination. — Paul Saunders, *Edward Jenner: The Cheltenham Years, 1795–1823* (Hanover, N.H.: University Press of New England, 1982), pp. 62, 147.

4. Cow Pox.

5. Chester was only twenty miles from Downing.

17. To Dr. Caleb Hillier Parry, Circus, Bath, 10 January 1805

Berkeley, January 10th 1805

Dear Parry[1]

When you can spare five minutes pray take your Pen & tell me when matters are likely to come to a conclusion between P. & the Parties in G.S.[2] — Since my return from Cheltenham, I have had a pretty close correspondence with P. but to no purpose; it began & ended in sparring. He is one of those very extraordinary Beings who never committed an error. In future I shall request H.[3] to be his Correspondent — I have done. Many a good Ream of Paper have I consumed in these fruitless attempts to render the Concern productive, by regulating his conduct.

I was much pleased at seeing a few days ago in the Bath, & some of the London Papers, the spirited resolutions of your County for the extermination of the Smallpox.[4] The conduct of Mr. Hobhouse on this occasion was of course peculiarly agreeable to me. You could not have found a more able Chairman. This irritable Flesh of mine, which you know so long smarted with sores, is now completely heal'd by the Balsam he pour'd over them on that day. If you should chance to see Mr. H. pray tell him this.

A neighbour of mine died yesterday from a disease of the Heart, which followed two or three severe attacks of accute Rheumatism. You may probably remember a Paper of mine that was given into the *Fleece Med: Socy.* on this Subject.[5] This & my other Papers are in your possession. If you would be good enough to convey them to me, I should be extremely happy in regaining them; particularly that I now allude to, as I am confident many a life is lost by not shielding the Heart at the going off of accute Rheumatism, which not unfrequently at that time feels a morbid determination of Blood. — Think of this request if you can & that on the first Page of my Letter. Is Dr. Charles Parry[6] at home? My respects to him, to Mrs. P. & your wide Circle.

Yours truly

E. Jenner

PS.   Can you recollect how long it is since you first heard me mention the idea of inoculating human Subjects with Vaccine Matter?

1. See Letters 1, 14, and 57.

The third paragraph of this letter was published in Jacobs, "Edward Jenner," p. 746.

2. George Pearson, M.D. (1751-1828), was an inoculator at the Vaccine Pock Institution in Golden Square. Although he had been originally one of Jenner's most active supporters, he now argued that Jenner's alleged, harmless cowpox disease did not exist, for he had obtained pustules resembling those of smallpox. This was because he and William Woodville had contaminated their cowpox matter with that of smallpox. See Jenner's "Letter on the Vaccine Inoculation," *Medical and Physical Journal* 3 (February 1800): 101-2. Pearson also testified against Jenner at the House of Commons investigation and continued to try to refute his claims. See Letter 8, n. 3.

3. Henry Jenner, his nephew, who had become his apprentice in 1783 and now assisted with Jenner's busy practice.

4. On 1 January 1805 the Royal Somerset Jennerian Society had been organized at Bath with Benjamin Hobhouse, M.P. (1757-1831), as chairman. His wife was Parry's sister. The society's purpose was to raise funds in order to carry on universal vaccination in the county. For reports see *Medical and Physical Journal* 13 (1805): 186-88, and 14 (1805): 348-53.

5. The Fleece Medical Society, which Jenner was instrumental in founding in May 1788, consisted of the following physicians and surgeons: John Heathfield Hickes, M.D., of Gloucester (later at Bristol); Edward Jenner; Thomas Paytherus of Ross; Daniel Ludlow, Jr., of Sodbury; and Caleb Hillier Parry, M.D., of Bath. They met at the Fleece Inn in Rodborough. On 29 July 1789 Jenner delivered a paper with the title "Remarks on a Disease of the Heart Following Acute Rheumatism, Illustrated by Dissections," which is evidently referred to in this letter. It was never published, and the manuscript has never been found. See Harry Keil, "A Note on Edward Jenner's Lost Manuscript on 'Rheumatism of the Heart,'" *Bulletin of the History of Medicine* 7 (1939): 409-11, and LeFanu, pp. 16-19.

6. Charles Henry Parry (1779-1860) was Caleb Hillier Parry's son. An Edinburgh M.D. in 1804, he had studied medicine at Göttingen in 1799 and traveled in Germany with Samuel Taylor Coleridge.

18.   To the Reverend Thomas Frognall Dibdin, Terrace, Kensington, 4 February [1805]

Many thanks to you, my dear Friend,[1] for your ready acquiescence in accepting the Post I suggested to you. I fear the Pages which this accompanies, will hardly reach the Terrace in time for the inspection of P.,[2] and yet I could have wish'd for it; for if it passes his double Eyes, it passes an ordeal indeed. It is with great regret I hear him even hint at leaving Cheltenham, & in my Letter to him there, I have said the moment he is off the following little Billet will be fixt upon my door "To be sold." There is a great dearth of mind in this place, Cheltenham; & no vast abundance of that sweet commodity friendship.

With respect to the Pamphlet, deal with it as if it were your own. I once thought of a quarto form, but now think it is long enough for the common shape; that is, if the Letter fixt upon be large enough to give it proper size. Let us have decent Paper. But the Printer — who shall be the Man? As I so much wish for secrecy, this will require your attention. If in its perusal, you should discover omissions of the names of any Men of consequence who have figured on the Vaccine side, pray give them to me. With respect to those which should be printed complete or incomplete, I must leave it in some measure to you. That you may correctly know whom I mean I shall send you in time the names at full length of all those whose initials only now appear, or whose names are abbreviated. But after all, if you should think it does not return a fair answer to the question of *cui bono?* candidly say so; and the sooner I hear your decision the better.

I am most truly pleas'd to find that Fortune has pencil'd down your name in her Memorandum Book, and most sincerely hope she may never rub it out till the object of your wishes be completely accomplish'd.

Adieu my dear Sir   Yours truly

E J.

As I shall be under some anxiety about the Parcel, you will indulge me much in sending a line when it arrives.

Monday Morning, 4th February [Cheltenham]

PS.   Manning,[3] whose direction you will see, has been here to take my Bust. He is a young Artist of merit & the Prime Conductor of Bacon's Works.[4] — If you should be strolling towards Warren St. give a look at it. —

I shall have a short Postscript for Moseley who is just out with a Pamphlet that merits the severest reproach.[5] Pray see it — It is quite diabolical.

The Names are sent — When writing I thought there would not have been time for it.

1. Thomas Frognall Dibdin, D.D. (1776–1847), a bibliographer characterized in the *DNB* as "an ignorant pretender, without the learning of a schoolboy, who published a quantity of books swarming with error of every description," had probably been recommended to Jenner by his close friend from Cheltenham, Thomas Pruen, to prepare Jenner's anonymous pamphlet for publication. The identity of the pamphlet to which Jenner is referring is unknown.

2. Thomas Pruen (ca. 1772–1834) was one of Jenner's close friends to whom Jenner wrote seventy-four letters preserved at the Wellcome Historical Medical Library. His literary interests had stimulated Dibdin to become a bibliophile, and in the latter's *Reminiscences of a Literary Life* (2 vols. [London, 1836], 1:158, 200–202) he wrote that Pruen, John Ring, and Jenner had induced him to write a poem in blank verse called "Vaccinia." After Jenner's death Pruen expected to become Jenner's biographer. See Letters 54 and A-15.

3. Charles Manning (1776–1812), who came from a family of sculptors. Jenner's bust was

exhibited at the Royal Academy. Manning's most famous work was the national monument in St. Paul's Cathedral to Captain George Hardinge, 1808. — Rupert Gunnis, *Dictionary of British Sculptors, 1660–1851* (London: Odhams Press, 1953), pp. 251–52.

4. John Bacon the Younger (1777–1859), successor to his more famous father, was probably the most prolific British sculptor in the early decades of the nineteenth century. See Gunnis, *Dictionary of British Sculptors,* pp. 28–32.

5. Benjamin Moseley, M.D. (d. 1819), surgeon-general of Jamaica for a number of years, received his medical degree from St. Andrews in 1784. He served as physician to Chelsea Hospital for more than thirty years. From the beginning, Moseley was a violent antivaccinationist. His *Treatise on the Lues Bovilla; or, The Cow Pox* was announced in the February 1805 issue of the *Gentleman's Magazine* (75, pt. 1:152).

19. To Edward Jones, Esq., Surgeon, Brinderwyn Hall, Montgomeryshire, 7 December 1805

Cheltenham — Glostershire
December 7th 1805

Dear Sir[1]

Permit me to present to you my best acknowledgements for your very excellent vindication of the practice of Vaccination,[2] which I had the pleasure of receiving a short time since from a Gentleman at Worcester. Having never met with anything better calculated to excite contempt for the malignant efforts of those who have attempted to delude the people and bring the new practice into discredit, I cannot but regret its being within the narrow circle of a few Friends. In my opinion, it should know no bounds, and therefore trust you will either put it into the hands of some London Bookseller yourself for republication, or allow me to do it; as I should feel quite happy in your granting me permission to suffer the expence to fall on me.[3]

I have taken the liberty of ordering my Bookseller in Town to send you Rowley's[4] & some other Pamphlets. If you should not deem Rowley too contemptible, a concise answer in the same animated style in which you attack Squirrel,[5] would be well received by the Public, & be productive of beneficial consequences; for there are heads so soft, that even such flimsy stuff as this makes impressions upon them.

I hope to be indulged with a line from you when convenient, and remain
Dear Sir   Your highly obliged   & very faithful Servant

Edwd. Jenner

PS.   Since writing the above I have seen the Gentleman's Magazine for the present Month. If you should chance to see it, you will find that Moseley[6] has far outstripp'd his Competitors in antivaccine fame, Squirrel, Birch[7] &

Rowley. I thought in point of scurrility, malevolence and misrepresentation, they had gone pretty great lengths, but Moseley has far surpass'd them.

1. Edward Jones was a member of the Royal College of Surgeons and surgeon to the Montgomeryshire Volunteer Legion. See also Letters 24, 30, and 84.

2. Jenner undoubtedly is referring to the pamphlet by Edward Jones, *Vaccination Vindicated against Misrepresentation and Calumny, in a Letter to his Patients* (Welshpool: J. Waidson, 1805).

3. There is no evidence that a London reprint was ever made.

4. William Rowley, *Cow-Pox Inoculation no Security against Small-Pox Infection*, 2nd ed. (London, 1805). Rowley (1743–1806) obtained his M.D. from St. Andrews, and was physician to the Marylebone Infirmary and consulting physician to the Queen's Lying-in Hospital. For a very uncomplimentary note on his life and literary creations see Munk, *Roll*, 2:340–42.

5. R. Squirrel, M.D. (whose real name was John Gale Jones), former resident apothecary to the Small-pox and Inoculation Hospital, had published *Observations addressed to the Public in general on Cow-Pox, shewing that it originates in Scrophula* (London, 1805).

6. Jenner is probably referring to "Dr. Moseley's Objections to Vaccination," *Gent. Mag.* 75, pt. 2 (1805): 897–901. There was a prolonged controversy in the form of letters to "Mr. Urban," the editor in the pages of the *Gentleman's Magazine* for a number of years. See also Letter 18, n. 5.

Jenner's staunch friend, John Ring, wrote a book against Moseley, *An Answer to Dr. Moseley, containing a Defence of Vaccination* (London, 1805), a copy of which was sent to Edward Jones by Jenner in January 1806, shortly after this letter was written. The inscribed copy is in the Henry Barton Jacobs Collection, Welch Medical Library.

7. John Birch, surgeon to St. Thomas's Hospital, had published "A Letter occasioned by the many Failures of Cow-Pox," in [W. R. Rogers], *An Examination of that Part of the Evidence relative to Cow-Pox, which was delivered to the Committee of the House of Commons*, 2nd. ed. (London, 1805). Another antivaccination publication was George Lipscomb, *A Dissertation of the Failure and Mischiefs of the Disease called the Cow-Pox* (London, 1805).

20. To Richard Phillips, New Bridge St., Black Friars Bridge, London, 23 February 1806

Cheltenham
Feb. 23, 1806

My dear Sir[1]

I have always an immense Pile of Letters before me unanswer'd; not thro' indolence but necessity — From this Pile, I this morning drew yours. Believe me I had not the most distant conception, however great your inclination & complete your powers, that you could have found time to abstract your thoughts from your ordinary engagements & direct them in the manner you have to the subject of Vaccination.[2] Accept my best thanks. You certainly set the venom flowing freely from the jaws of that mad animal M — —.[3] I was sorry to see it spread so thickly over the Pages of a

Magazine,[4] that once was thought an ornament in the Library of a Gentleman.

I will now submit to your consideration a subject that may prove both useful & interesting. In the Med: & Phys: Journal there are a great number of very excellent Papers relating to the subject of Vaccination. There they lie, as it were entomb'd, as far as regards the public Eye. This Publication being entirely medical, meets the medical Eye only, or at least with exceptions of no great consequence. What think you? At the present hour when the arch Impostor Moseley & his Dupes, Rowley, Squirrel & the rest,[5] have so deluded the Metropolis, might not these Papers be easily form'd into a Volume that would be gladly received, & be absolutely new to the Public in general?[6] When you have had time to give this a thought, pray favor me with a line.

Your very faithful & obedient Servant

Edw: Jenner

1. Richard Phillips (1767–1840), publisher of the *Monthly Magazine*. A friend of Joseph Priestley and a man of radical political views, he had been imprisoned for eighteen months in 1793 for selling Thomas Paine's *Rights of Man*. He published cheap literature on many subjects for popular instruction.

2. In his "Half-Yearly Retrospect of Domestic Literature," published in a supplementary number of the *Monthly Magazine* (20 [January 1806]: 603–5), Phillips had reviewed the literature on the vaccine controversy. He also published at least one book in favor of vaccination: Robert Willan, *On Vaccine Inoculation* (London, 1806).

3. See Letter 18, n. 4 and Letter 19, n. 6, which describe Benjamin Moseley's antivaccination activities.

4. Letters by Joseph Roberts and Benjamin Moseley were published in *Gent. Mag.* 76, pt. 1 (January 1806): 25–27.

5. See Letter 19.

6. There is no evidence that this suggestion was carried out.

21. To [Dr. Alexander J. G. Marcet, 30 June 1806]

My dear Sir[1]

I am much obliged to you for making me acquainted with your intelligent Friend Dr. Willemoes.[2] He has promised to breakfast with me to morrow at nine — Would it be possible for You to meet him? I should be happy to see you. This young man could communicate a Fact to me which would at this time be peculiarly interesting. At the time he left Copenhagen, it seems, the Smallpox was subdued by the powers of the Cowpox! On Wednesday the Chancellor of the Excheq'r.[3] will bring forward a motion on the subject of Vaccination. Some Papers will be put into his hands *to morrow* at 12 o'clock. If among them was a Letter, stating that you had seen Dr. Willemoes who communicated the fact; or, if you please, signify to him in what manner he should state it himself, it would prove of considerable consequence to me & my cause. Pardon, I pray you, this hasty suggestion & believe me   truly Yours

27 Gt. Russel St.   Edw: Jenner

Monday Evening[4]

PS.   If it be impossible to give me a Letter on this subject to morrow, I would endeavor to get [it] into Lord Henry Petty's hands on Wednesday morning. — The Population of Copenhagen should be stated.

1. See Letter 7, n. 1.
2. Probably Frederick Wilhelm Willemoes (1778–?), a graduate of the University of Copenhagen in 1803.   — Adolph Carl Peter Callisen, *Medicinisches Schriftsteller-Lexicon,* 33 vols. (Copenhagen, 1835), 21:195.
3. Lord Henry Petty. Jenner's friends felt that he had not been sufficiently rewarded by his parliamentary grant of £10,000 in 1802. Therefore on 2 July 1806 Petty brought the business of vaccination again before the House of Commons. He recommended that the Royal College of Physicians draw up a report of its opinion on the value of vaccination. For an account of the parliamentary proceedings see James Moore, *The History and Practice of Vaccination* (London, 1817), pp. 175 ff.; Baron, *Life,* 2:56 ff.; and *Report of The Royal College of Physicians of London, on Vaccination,* ordered to be printed, by the House of Commons, 8 July 1807 (London, 1807). Jenner was awarded an additional £20,000.
4. The date "30 June 1806" was written in another hand in the upper corner of the letter.

22.   To — — —, 30 August 1806

My dear Madam[1]

I had no conception when I had the pleasure of seeing you last, of being detain'd till this time in Town.[2] However here I am; but on Monday morning hope to take my departure for Berkeley & in a few days after, coming to Cheltenham.

You will pardon me I hope; but I could not forbear smiling at your simplicity in supposing such a Man as Moseley[3] would have had a trust of such importance reposed in him as to be placed at the head of the Medical Staff to the Expedition about to quit our Shores.

Lord Henry Petty spoke most charmingly in the House of Commons on the Vaccine Subject.[4] The Reports I continue to rec've from abroad are delightful. Among my last are these: that the smallpox is quite subdued in the City of Lyons; and at Geneva, there has not been a Small pox Funeral these five years. While Alas! in London & its Environs the smallest computation is six thousand within the last twelve months!! Bravo, Drs. Moseley, Squirrel, Lipscombe & Co.[5]

The Parliamentary business, I fear, will bring me to Town early in the Winter.

I hope you are enjoying the sweets of the Country — Not one word has reach'd me since I saw you respecting Mrs. Watts. It was impossible for me to call upon her, when I found on my arrival in Town She associated with such Persons as some of those I have just named.

Believe me dear Madam   with great esteem   Yours very faithfully

E Jenner

Gt. Russel St.

Friday 30 August 1806

1. Probably a Cheltenham acquaintance. The third paragraph was published in Miller, "Letters," p. 13.
2. London.
3. See Letter 18, n. 4.
4. See Letter 21, n. 3. There is a detailed report in "British and Foreign History for the Year 1806," *New Annual Register . . . for the Year 1806* (London, 1807), pt. 1, pp. 221–23.
5. See Letter 19.

23.   To Dr. Alexander J. G. Marcet, St. Mary Axe., London, 21 November 1806

My dear Sir[1]

I am extremely obliged to you for your Communications. Your materials for the College are of the choicest kind — Pray lay them before that learned Body.[2] I cannot now put my hand upon the Letter you procured for me from your Danish Friend;[3] but you must remember, I presume, the most interesting parts of it. It is, I believe, with my Papers at Berkeley. The Report from Lyons must be very important. A sight of it, would certainly be very gratifying to me, if it is not too long for you to transcribe. A few days since, I rec'd from Madrid a Document respecting Vaccination which fills me with more astonishment than anything that has yet reach'd me on that subject. It comes in the form of "Suplemento a la Gazeta de Madrid."[4] I shall get it reprinted,[5] & contrive to send you a Copy; therefore I will not now anticipate the contents of this very singular paper. Would to Heaven the British Cabinet had shewn the same Philanthropic Spirit as that of Spain!

I had not heard of Mr. Duvillard's Work[6] till you mention'd it. Do you conceive it to be anything like a popular work sent out a few years since by Malthus?[7]

Poor Swann![8] I was shock'd at the alarming accounts I repeatedly heard respecting his health; but a few days ago we had intelligence of an opposite nature. Barwis[9] tells us the pain was much abated and he began to sleep — But still I fear the case is of a formidable nature. Walker[10] will be troublesome to our Society as long as he lives. I have just heard some odd Anecdotes of this versatile Genius from a Gentleman of Bristol, at which City, he once exhibited as a public Lecturer on Astronomy. I wish his Eyes had still been directed towards the Stars, & that he had not bent them downwards to disturb the peace of the *Jennerians.*

I fear it will not be in my power to get a Paper ready on any subject for the 1st Vol: of the Medical Society.[11] The business preparing for Parliament occasions at this time an increase of correspondence. But on a future day, you shall find me punctual to my promise. Have you seen the last number of the Med: & Chirurgical Review?[12] The logical deductions from my Letters to Willan are the most absurd than [*sic*] can be conceived, and shew what slender Twigs the antivaccinists are now catching at. I think they must find a complete overthrow in the pages of the Edinburgh Review for October[13] — Moseley and his Coadjutors are lash'd most severely. I hope Mrs. Marcet has by this time forgotten there is such a thing as a Nerve. Mrs. Jenner unites in best wishes   with Yours very truly

Cheltenham 21 Novr. 1806   Edwd. Jenner

There is no hot Spring here.[14]

PS.   Extract of a Letter from a Surgeon at Portsea Hants —
"I am sorry to say that Mr. Hobbs of this Town has lately lost an only Child in the Smallpox inoculated by Mr. Goldson"[15]

1. See Letter 7, n. 1.

2. The Royal College of Physicians of London was carrying on its investigation on the value of vaccination. See Letter 21.

3. See Letter 21, n. 2.

4. Jenner is undoubtedly referring to the report in the *Gaceta de Madrid,* 14 October 1806, which describes the successful outcome of the expedition sent out by the king of Spain under Dr. Francisco Xavier Balmis to bring vaccination to the Spanish possessions in the New World. For a detailed account of the expedition's work see S. F. Cook, "Francisco Xavier Balmis and the Introduction of Vaccination to Latin America," *Bulletin of the History of Medicine* 11 (1942):543–60; ibid. 12:70–101; and M. M. Smith, *The "Real Expedición Marítima de la Vacuna" in New Spain and Guatemala* (Philadelphia: American Philosophical Society, 1974).

5. The report of the Balmis expedition was published in the *Medical and Physical Journal* 17 (1807): 12–16, and in the *Monthly Magazine* 23 (February 1807): 38–40.

6. Emmanuel-Etienne Duvillard de Durand, *Analyse et tableaux de l'influence de la petite vérole sur la mortalité à chaque âge, et de celle qu'un préservatif tel que la vaccine peut avoir sur la population et la longévité* (Paris, 1806). Duvillard de Durand (1755–1832) was a mathematician who pioneered in France the application of the calculus of probability to political and social questions. From 1786 on, he attempted to create life insurance, still unknown in France, and wrote a lengthy work which he presented to the Académie des sciences in 1796. The only part published was the book cited above. In 1807 he published *Rapport du Collège des médecins de Londres sur la vaccination, suivi d'une analyse de son influence sur la mortalité et la population.* — *Dictionnaire de Biographie Française* (Paris, 1970), 12:1061–62.

7. Malthus's *Essay on the Principle of Population* (London, 1798).

8. John Swann died on 6 February 1807, according to the *Gentleman's Magazine,* "in his 39th year, . . . an eminent paper-maker at Wolvercott, near Oxford," — *Gent. Mag.,* 1807, pt. 2, p. 181.

9. See Letter 6.

10. John Walker (1759–1830) was resident inoculator and medical secretary of the Royal Jennerian Society from its founding in 1803 till the summer of 1806, when he resigned because of internal animosities and disagreements about how to carry out the campaign for vaccination. —John Epps, *The Life of John Walker, M.D.,* 2nd ed. (London, 1832), pp. 88 ff. For a view of Walker's activities written by one of his opponents, see James Moore, *The History and Practice of Vaccination* (London, 1817), pp. 211 ff. Moore pointed out that the adversaries were divided according to their religious professions: Walker, being a Quaker, was supported by his Quaker brethren, as against the Anglicans, Dissenters, and Freethinkers, who wished to depose him. Speaking of Walker's Quaker friends, Moore wrote, "At all general meetings their broad-brimmed hats shaded the boards; for their schismatic assiduity was most conspicuous, though their primitive meekness was indiscernible. In support of their friend, they argued slily, wrangled tumultously, and voted almost unanimously."

11. Marcet and John Yelloly had founded in 1805 a new society, the Medical and Chirurgical Society of London. Their portraits today are at the Royal Society of Medicine in London. The first volume of the society's publication, *Medico-Chirurgical Transactions* (1809), included two papers by Jenner: "Observations on the Distemper of Dogs" (pp. 263–68) and "Two Cases of Small-pox Infection communicated to the Foetus in utero under peculiar Circumstances: with additional remarks" (pp. 269–75).

12. *Medical and Chirurgical Review* 13 (1806): 300–313, where Robert Willan's book *On Vaccine Inoculation* (London, 1806) was reviewed. Pp. i–viii, appendix 1, of Willan's book printed part of a letter from Jenner to Willan, dated 23 February 1806.

13. *The Edinburgh Review* 9 (1807): 32–66, begins with the following statement: "Medical subjects ought in general, we think, to be left to the Medical Journals; but the question as to the efficacy of vaccination is of such incalculable importance, and of such universal interest, as to excuse a little breach of privilege." The following books were then reviewed: Robert Willan, *On Vaccine Inoculation* (London, 1806); Benjamin Moseley, *Commentaries on the Lues Bovilla, or Cow-Pox,* 2nd ed. (London, 1806); James Moore, *A Reply to the Antivaccinists* (London, 1806); and Robert Squirrel, *Observations on the pernicious Consequences of Cow-Pox Inoculation, containing many well authenticated Cases, proving its insecurity against the Small-Pox,* 2nd ed. (London, 1806).

14. "The alkaline-saline mineral waters at Cheltenham, discovered in 1716, are valuable

for their diuretic effect and as a stimulant to the liver." — L. Russell Muirhead, ed., *The Blue Guides: England,* 5th ed. (London: Ernest Benn, 1950), p. 229. See Jenner's description in Letter 56.

15. Jenner and his followers were attempting to suppress inoculation of smallpox, which had become widely accepted in England.

24. To Edward Jones, Esq., Welch Pool, Montgomeryshire, 13 December 1806

My dear Sir[1]

I presume you have seen the Address of the College of Physicians to the Faculty throughout the British Realms, requesting them to lay before them their evidence, & to give their opinions on the subject of Vaccination. From an intimation lately received from Town, I have reason to think the College wish soon to make up their report for Parliament.[2] Your information will be valuable — You will therefore excuse the liberty I take in hinting to you the necessity for its being sent *soon.*

You need not be told, how greatly you have already obliged me, by addressing to the Public your excellent Pamphlet in favor of Vaccination,[3] & how sincerely I am

dear Sir, Yours

Edwd. Jenner

Cheltenham
Decr. 13 1806

Lest you should not have seen the Advertisement of the College, I will send you a Copy of it.

I should be much pleased with a line from you. Pray do me the favor to accept the enclos'd[4] — You will be much gratified at the perusal of this glorious narrative — I cannot but regret that such an enterprize had not been atchiev'd by the British Nation.

[In another hand on the third page of Jenner's letter:]

His Majesty has been graciously pleased, in compliance with an address from the honourable House of Commons, to direct his Royal College of Physicians in London to enquire into the present state of Vaccination in the United Kingdom; to report their observations and opinion upon the practice, and the Evidence adduced in its support, and upon the causes which have hitherto retarded its general adoption.

The College are now engaged in the investigation of the several questions thus referred to them, and give this public notice they are ready to receive in[formation] upon the Subject of Vaccination, from Medical [Practi]tioners, as to the result of their Exper[   ]a[   ]vils.

[   ] Letters to be addressed to the Register of [   ] Royal College of Physicians, under cove[   ] Spencer[5] Secretary of States' Office, London

Jas Hervey[6]

Novr. 20th 1806

Register.

1. See Letters 19, 30, and 84.
2. See Letter 21, n. 3.
3. See Letter 19, n. 2.
4. Probably a copy of the article describing the Balmis expedition. See Letter 23, n. 4.
5. George John Spencer, second Earl Spencer (1758–1834) was home secretary in 1806-7.
6. James Hervey, M.D. (d. 1824), was registrar of the college from 1784 to 1814. He was also the first registrar of the National Vaccine Establishment.

25. To Dr. Alexander J. G. Marcet, at Swann's Esq., Woolvercott near Oxford, 13 December 1806

My dear Sir[1]

I have not time to answer your Letter by return of Post, but only just sufficient to thank you for it; and to request it as a great favor that you will immediately give me a line from Woolvercott. I fear your communication will be the reverse of what I could wish to hear of my excellent Friend, poor Swann.[2]

When you wrote, it is clear you had not rec'd a Packet I sent to Town Saturday last, with many others to be put into the 2d Post. It contain'd a most valuable Document on the Vaccine Subject from Madrid.[3]

That your efforts to restore poor Swann may be attended with the success we wish prays your sincere Friend & Servant

E Jenner

PS. Give S. my best wishes, & Barwis[4] if he is at Woolvercott.

There is no warm Spring discover'd here[5] — This notion must have arisen from Thompson's making Hot Baths in his Field.

Cheltenham

Wednesday afternoon near 4 o'clock [*Postal date:* Dec. 13, 1806]

1. See Letter 7, n. 1. This letter was redirected to 51 St. Mary Axe, Leaden Hall St.
2. See Letter 23, n. 8. Marcet was evidently Swann's physician.
3. See Letter 23, n. 4.
4. See Letter 6.
5. See Letter 23, n. 14.

26. To Mr. Richens, Esq., Asst. Surgeon, Royal Artillery, Exeter, 18 December 1806

Sir[1]   Cheltenham   18th December 1806

Your Letter of Decr. 10th directed to me in London has just reach'd me at this place. It shall be immediately forwarded to the Institution,[2] and I doubt not that you will be very quickly supplied with Vaccine Matter. I will just take the liberty of mentioning, that among your Men, it may be prudent to produce more Pustules than one — not that one is not sufficient to protect a Person from the Smallpox, but among those who labor, accidents are very liable to happen which interrupt it in its ordinary progress; on which so much depends. To guard against accidents of this nature, I now commonly make two or three Punctures.

You have seen I presume a Paper of mine on the subject of Herpetic Eruptions shewing their interference with the progress of the Vaccine Pustule. It may be found in the Medical & Phys: Journal for August 1804.[3]

I am Sir   Your obedient humble Servant

Edw: Jenner

1. The recipient of this letter cannot be identified beyond the information found in the address.
2. The Royal Jennerian Society. Jenner also refers to it as the Royal Jennerian Institution in Letter 13.
3. *Medical and Physical Journal* 12 (1804): 97–102. (LeFanu 79.)

27. To the Reverend George Charles Jenner, [1806 or 1821]

Dear George[1]

The weather at present looks promising for a fine day to morrow, & I most ardently hope nothing will prevent your giving me enough of your company to go into a careful perusal of the Pamphlet with me.

I do assure you, had I been aware of the great anxiety it would have occasion'd, I never would have sent a page to the Press on the subject of artificial Eruptions[2] — You have felt their smart upon the skin, but I upon my Brain.

Come to breakfast if you can, & make no promises about returning.

Most truly Yours

E Jenner

Thursday Afternoon

1. The Reverend George Charles Jenner, son of Edward Jenner's elder brother Henry, was both a physician and a clergyman, and helped Jenner with his publications. In 1801 he had published a letter supporting vaccination (LeFanu 143), and in 1805 he had published the Parliamentary proceedings relative to vaccination (Letter 13, n. 4). See also Letters 98 and 99.

2. Jenner was evidently in the process of republishing the paper on herpetic eruptions mentioned in Letter 26. It appeared as *On the Varieties and Modifications of the Vaccine Pustule, Occasioned by an Herpetic State of the Skin* (Cheltenham: H. Ruff, 1806). (LeFanu 81.)

Early in 1822 Jenner published, with many editorial difficulties described in Letter 90, *A Letter to Charles Henry Parry . . . on the Influence of Artificial Eruptions* (LeFanu 109), which provides an alternate possible date of late 1821 for this letter.

28. To Samuel Bell Labatt, M.D., Dublin, 11 February 1807

Berkeley Glostre.

Dear Sir[1]   Feb: 11 1807

I have this evening been favor'd with your obliging Letter enclosing the Report of the Progress of the Cow-Pock Institution in Dublin.[2]

Be assured it is a gratification of the highest kind to hear that the practice goes on so successfully. I must request you to present my respectful Comps. to the Gentlemen of the Institution & to accept the best wishes of Dear Sir,

Your obliged & very faithful   Humble Servant

E Jenner

To S. B. Labatt M.D. Dublin

1. Samuel Bell Labatt, M.D., Edinburgh 1797, was in 1802 made licentiate of the King and Queen's College of Physicians of Ireland. He served from 1814 to 1821 as master of the Dublin Lying-In Hospital. — Adolph Carl Peter Callisen, *Medicinisches Schriftsteller-Lexicon,* 33 vols. (Copenhagen, 1835), 10:474, and T. Percy C. Kirkpatrick, *The Book of the Rotunda Hospital* (London: Bartholomew Press, 1913). Labatt published *An Address to the Medical Practitioners of Ireland, on the Subject of Cow-Pock* (Dublin: Gilbert and Hodges, 1805).

This letter was published in Hamilton Labatt, *Letters addressed by Edward Jenner, M.D. to the late Samuel Bell Labatt, M.D. of Dublin, on the Subject of Vaccination* (Dublin: M. H. Gill, 1859), reprinted from the *Dublin Quarterly Journal of Medical Science,* vol. 27 (1859), and was reproduced photographically in Miller, "Letters," p. 16.

2. The Cow-Pock Institution in Dublin was established in 1804 under the patronage of Lord Hardwicke. Dr. Labatt was secretary and inoculator. — *Report of The Royal College of Physicians of London, on Vaccination* (London, 1807), p. 9. Hardwicke, a Cheltenham friend who became lord lieutenant of Ireland, had written to Jenner in February 1803 for guidance in establishing vaccination in Ireland. — LeFanu, p. 68; Paul Saunders, *Edward Jenner: The Cheltenham Years, 1795–1823* (Hanover, N.H.: University Press of New England, 1982), pp. 130–31, 146.

29. To Miss Bignell, [London, March 1807]

My dear Madam[1]

I fully intended calling in Montague St. this morning, had I not been made acquainted with Mrs. Mayow's wishes.

Pray present my Comps. & say I shall be there about twelve.

Truly yours

E Jenner

I have a Friend here who wishes to see Stuart's Pamphlet.[2]

1. Miss Bignell lived at Sydenham, near London, and like Mrs. Pennant (Letter 16) was carrying on vaccination. — Ludwig Darmstaedter, "Ein Brief von Edward Jenner vom 12. VIII 1805," *Deutsche Medizinische Wochenschrift* 52 (1926): 1350.

2. Probably *A Letter to Lord Henry Petty on Coercive Vaccination* (London, 1807), by John Ferdinand Smyth Stuart (1745–1814). This was a violent diatribe against vaccination. A frontispiece shows Jenner adorned with a tail and hoofs, feeding basketsful of infants to a hideous monster. Jenner is described as follows: "A mighty and horrible monster, with the horns of a bull, the hind hoofs of a horse, the jaws of the kraken, the teeth and claws of a tiger, the tail of a cow, — all the evils of Pandora's box in his belly, — plague, pestilence, leprosy, purple blotches, fetid ulcers, and filthy sores, covering his body, — and an atmosphere of accumulated disease, pain, and death around him, has made his appearance in the world, and devours mankind, — especially poor, helpless infants; not by scores only, or hundreds, or thousands, but by hundreds of thousands." This description was republished in a section entitled "Vaccination, and Its Opponents" in R. Chambers, ed., *The Book of Days: A Miscellany of Popular Antiquities in Connection with the Calendar,* 2 vols. (London and Edinburgh, 1869), 1:628.

Stuart was an American Loyalist who had studied medicine in Edinburgh, emigrated to Virginia, and set up his practice near Williamsburg. When the War for Independence began, he was forced to leave and joined the British forces. He returned to England at the end of the war.

30. To Edward Jones, Esq., Dalforwin Hall, Montgomeryshire, 16 July 1807

My dear Sir[1]

I had no conception I should have any difficulty in obtaining your Diploma, but the precision that marks the Scotch character it seems, calls for an obedience to the exact complyance to the form of the Certificate they have laid down at St. Andrews.[2] Can you point out to me any Physician here who is *personally* acquainted with you. Here stands the impediment at present. Dr. Willan, whose note I enclose, sticks at this point, & so will others, unless they can certify that they are personally acquainted with you.[3] As for myself, I chuse to put a *figurative* meaning to the expression, and feel myself sufficiently satisfied from the intercourse I have had with you that you are justly entitled to the degree of Doctor of Physic from any University. I shall be ready to join my name with any Physician in your own neighbourhood if you will send back the Certificate; but if you could make it convenient to visit London the business could be executed at once; and I can assure you with truth I should be very happy to see you.

Believe me, dear Sir,   very truly yours

E Jenner

Bedford Place [London]
July 16 1807

PS.   Pardon this short Letter; I am always interrupted when I attempt to write in Town.

1. See Letter 19. Other Jones letters are nos. 24 and 84. All but the last sentence of this letter has been published in Miller, "Letters," p. 9.
2. During the eighteenth century the Scottish universities began the practice of granting degrees in medicine *in absentia* to candidates who had never attended the university but presented testimonials of their knowledge from prominent physicians. At St. Andrews the custom was extensive: at the end of the eighteenth century over nine-tenths of all degrees granted were in medicine, and most of these were *in absentia*. The following form was adopted in 1802 as a certificate for the two physicians who recommended candidates: "We, A.B., residing at . . . and C.D., residing at . . . do hereby certify that G.F., candidate for the degree of M.D., is a gentleman of respectable character, that he has received a liberal and classical education, that he has attended a complete course of lectures in the several branches of Medicine, and that from *personal knowledge* we judge him worthy of the honour of a doctor's degree in Medicine. Dated and signed A.B., M.D., and C.D., M.D." The system was condemned by the Royal Commission in 1830.   — *Votiva Tabella: A Memorial Volume of St. Andrews University* (Glasgow, 1911), pp. 213–14, 217–19.
   Jenner's own degree from St. Andrews was of this nature. He was recommended by his two friends J.H. Hickes, M.D., of Gloucester and Caleb Hillier Parry, M.D., of Bath.   — "Jenner Centenary Number," *British Medical Journal,* pt. 1 (23 May 1896), p. 1247.
3. Robert Willan (see Letter 23, n. 12) is chiefly remembered today for his work in dermatology. It appears that Jenner had wanted Willan to endorse Jones. Another sponsor must have eventually been found, since Letter 84, of 1818, is addressed to Dr. E. Jones.

31. Dr. Alexander J. G. Marcet, St. Mary Axe, London, 21 July 1807

My dear Sir[1]

I beg your acceptance of a Copy of *the Reports*[2] — that of the Col: of Phys: is as warm as I could expect; & perhaps it will prove more impressive than opinions deliver'd in a more energetic Form — But what cold, icy-hearted Mortal drew up the Report of the Col: of Surgeons (not of Scotland or of Ireland) but of England?[3] How unfortunate, that a Body of Men so respectable should have suffer'd resentment thus to have operated. I shall hope to talk this over with you & our Friends to morrow evening. I really think it will be necessary to publish the Report (for which I have the Speaker's leave) with a Commentary.

Truly yours

E Jenner

PS. Your Letters are arrived & the elegant Drawing of Mrs. M.[4] — a thousand thanks to her — I am not surpris'd at what your Friend the M.P. felt when he read the report of the Coll: of Surgeons. It *must* have an explanation & then what now appears frightful will appear in a state the very opposite. Mark the small number of Eruptive Cases — this proves what I have stated that Vaccination tends to destroy the disposition to eruptions & not to excite it — again — if 50,000 Children were scratch'd with a thorn one out of such a multitude might die in consequence.[5] Pray thank your Nephew for the great obligations he has confer'd upon me.

E J.

1. See Letter 7, n. 1, for references to the twenty-two letters to Marcet published herein. The first three sentences of this letter were published in Miller, "Letters," p. 14.

2. *Report of the Royal College of Physicians of London on Vaccination. With an Appendix, containing the Opinions of the Royal Colleges of Physicians of Edinburgh and Dublin; and of the Royal Colleges of Surgeons of London, of Dublin, and of Edinburgh* (London, 1807). Also published in *Medical and Physical Journal* 18 (1807): 97–111.

3. While the other medical organizations in the report endorsed vaccination enthusiastically, the report of the Royal College of Surgeons of London was a formal, matter-of-fact presentation of statistics based upon questionnaires sent out to its members, with no commentary or recommendations.

4. Mrs. Jane Marcet. See Letter 15, n. 6.

5. A reference to the statistics in the Royal College of Surgeons' report, wherein out of a total of 164,381 persons vaccinated, it was reported that there were 3 fatalities, 56 were later attacked by smallpox, 66 had eruptions of the skin, and 24 had inflammation of the arm.

32. To Dr. Alexander J. G. Marcet, St. Mary Axe, London, 18 August [1807]

My dear Friend[1]

I really feel distress'd at my inadvertency — From mistaking the Child for that Little one of yours whom I first vaccinated; & on inspecting the arm, finding the impression on the skin so unusually faint, I was somewhat confused, & fear some unguarded expressions might have dropp'd before I attempted to explain. Fine me how you please — You will let me off very easy by coming in to the following arrangement. Make my best Compliments to Mrs. Schmidtmeyer & tell her if she will do me the favor to bring the young Lady to Bedford Place on Thursday 12 o'Clock, a little one shall be ready to meet her with a Vaccine Pock in the highest state of perfection,[2] & that we can then remove every shadow of doubt respecting the present secur[ity].

With best regards to Mrs. Marcet   Yours most truly

E Jenner

Bedford Place [London]
Tuesday morning —

PS.   Are you aware that your history of the Case accounts for the faintness of the impression.

1. See Letter 7, n. 1, for references to the other Jenner-Marcet letters.
2. It is interesting to note that Jenner was performing arm-to-arm vaccination here. See his vaccination instructions in Letter 102.

33.   To John Ring, Esq., 17 December 1807

My dear Sir[1]

By yesterday's Coach I dispatch'd my Packets to Portsmouth. As time was running short, I thought there would be less risk of delay in sending it thus, than in consigning it to your care in Town. The Letters of introduction, were sent to Mr. Savage[2] by the Post, & I most sincerely hope they may prove useful to him. They were address'd to Dr. Russell & Mr. Shoolbred.[3] I hope he has taken some Copies of his Pamphlet respecting New Zealand.

Pray present my best wishes to Dr. Cabbell[4] & tell him your recommendation is sufficient to obtain for him any suffrage within my reach. When Murray sends me the Diplomas[5] (which did not arrive with the Papers of Instructions & the Reports) I could perhaps at the same time have a List of the Governors of St. George's Hospital.

Speaking of one of our Public Jennerian Papers, in a letter I lately rec'd from you, the old adage of "Too many Cooks &c" was brought in with much propriety. On perusing the Paper of Instructions,[6] I perceive the Proverb again applicable; & here I must confess myself one of the fraternity, or Co.

(the Firm I think consisted of Ring, Addington,[7] Merriman[8] & Jenner) engaged in cooking up this Dish. Many parts of it I fear will be unpalatable to the Public; I own it is to me, & I think you don't much relish it. I can't now point out all the unsavory parts but in a Letter to Murray which goes to Town by the same conveyance as this, I have shewn where some of the bad ingredients got into the Dish, which, to my taste, so much injured it. Pray had not a certain profess'd Cook in Th − − t Street, a finger in the Pie after the others had quitted it?

Adieu, my dear Friend − Yours most truly

Edw. Jenner

Cheltenham 17 Decr. 1807

PS. If you should find that the information you have rec'd respecting the Duke of Richmond be correct, you will have the kindness to let me know it & I will take care that his Grace shall know how shamefully he has been taken in by one of the greatest Knaves in England. With Mr. Blair's[9] permission I should have no objection to sign the Diplomas; but still I presume the signature of the President will be necessary as giving Dignity to the Thing −

1. John Ring (1752–1821), a London surgeon, was an early advocate of vaccination of whom Jenner wrote in 1815 as having performed the greatest number of vaccinations: "Think, my friend, on his vast losses in devoting so much time and expenditure to our cause." − Baron, *Life*, 2:395. In addition to a number of pamphlets defending vaccination, in 1803 he had joined Jenner in publishing the "Answer to Lord Hardwick's Letter," describing the best way to preserve vaccine matter, in *Medical and Physical Journal* 9 (1803): 541–42. (LeFanu 74.)

2. John Savage, surgeon, was setting out on a voyage to India from Portsmouth. He had recently published *Some Account of New Zealand, particularly the Bay of Islands and surrounding Country, with a Description of the Religion and Government, Language, Arts, Manufactures, Manners and Customs of the Natives, &c.* (London, 1807).

3. William Russell, surgeon, was the first superintendent general of vaccine inoculation to be appointed by the governor-general in Bengal. His duties were to provide a constant source of vaccine matter, to vaccinate native children, and to teach the Hindu and Moslem physicians how to vaccinate. Ill health forced him to leave Calcutta and return to England. His successor was John Shoolbred, who published in 1804 a *Report on the Progress of Vaccine Inoculation in Bengal, from the period of its introduction in November, 1802, to the end of the year 1803.*

4. Probably Joseph Carrington Cabell of Virginia, whose diary in the Alderman Library at the University of Virginia described conversations with Jenner in 1804. − LeFanu, p. 139.

5. Charles Murray, surgeon, was secretary to the board of directors of the Royal Jennerian Society. Members were given engraved diplomas.

6. A copy is preserved at the Wellcome Historical Medical Library, which possesses papers of the Royal Jennerian Society. See also Baron, *Life*, 2:361.

7. See Letter 12.

8. Samuel Merriman (1771–1852) had entered into the pamphlet warfare over vaccination, publishing *Observations on some late Attempts to depreciate the Value and Efficacy of Vaccine Inoculation* (London, 1805). He became a leading obstetrician and was physician-accoucheur to the Middlesex Hospital as well as to the Westminster General Dispensary.

9. William Blair (1766–1822), surgeon, was director of the Royal Jennerian Society and surgeon of the Lock Hospital. In 1806 he published *The Vaccine Contest*, a rebuttal to the efforts of William Rowley (see Letter 19, n. 4) to discredit vaccination. Later he published *Hints for the Consideration of Parliament, in a Letter to Dr. Jenner, on the supposed Failure of Vaccination at Ringwood; on the prevalent Abuse of variolous Inoculation, and on the Practice of the Smallpox Hospital* (London, 1808).

34. To Charles Murray, Esq., Bedford Row, London, [August 1808]

My dear Sir[1]

Dr. Knowles[2] tells me he thought a Board would be assembled on Monday next for receiving the Cambridge Report — I don't think it will be ready so soon.

I should be obliged to you for another peep at Dr. McKenzie's Report,[3] & pray don't forget to let me have the Ledger which you said contain'd the full particulars of a tale *amour extraordinary.*

Truly yours

Edw. Jenner

Russel St.

Thursday [August 1808]

1. Here and in the following letter Jenner is writing to Murray in his capacity as secretary to the board of directors of the Royal Jennerian Society, from which Walker had resigned as resident vaccinator in 1806. See also Letters 55, 58, and 62. Seventeen letters from Jenner to Murray, written between 1806 and 1817, are in the possession of the College of Physicians of Philadelphia. Eleven of these are published in S. Weir Mitchell, "The Manuscript Letters of Jenner in Possession of the College," *Transactions of the College of Physicians of Philadelphia*, 3rd ser. 22 (1900): 101–11.

2. Dr. James Sheridan Knowles (1784–1862) later became a well-known playwright and actor. After John Walker resigned as resident vaccinator of the Jennerian Society, Knowles, then only twenty-two, was appointed to the position. He had studied medicine under Dr. Robert Willan and purchased an M.D. from the University of Aberdeen.

3. A. M'Kenzie, M.D., was superintendent general of vaccine inoculation at Madras. His *General Abstract of Persons vaccinated at the Presidency of Madras, and at the subordinate Stations subject to the Authority of this Government, from the 1st of September, 1805, to the 31st of August, 1806* was published in the *Medical and Physical Journal* 17 (1807): 544–45, and also in the *Philadelphia Medical Museum* 4 (1808): 142–43.

35.　To Charles Murray, Esq., Bedford Row, London, October 1808

Pray look over the enclos'd & return it to me as soon as you can. I think one or two of our Resolutions respecting J.W.[1] should be copied from the Societies Books for his Grace's inspection. — Will you furnish me also with one or two of the circular Letters?

E.J.

1. John Walker. See Letter 23, n. 10.

36.　To Dr. Alexander J. G. Marcet, St. Mary Axe, London, [28 October 1808]

My dear Sir,[1]

You were good enough to call here a few days ago, I find, & leave some message about an Embassy going to Abyssinia. I cannot perfectly collect from my Servant what you suggested; but whatever it was, if you will have the goodness to explain, you shall find me attentive to it.

Still you see I am in Town; chain'd, as if were, by some magic Spell; but I trust it will soon be broken.

Pray make my best respects to Mrs. Marcett & believe me

Most truly yours

Edw. Jenner

Gt. Russel St.
Friday night [28 October 1808]

1. For the list of other Marcet letters see Letter 7, n. 1.

37.　To Dr. Alexander J. G. Marcet, Russell Square, London, 9 December 1808

Berkeley Glostershire
Decr. 9th 1808

My dear Friend[1]

Whenever I make a promise it is always my intention to perform it; but somehow or another, I am so ill fated as to break a great many. The delays which took place in gaining the expected information on the subject my Paper was intended to speak of, were vexatious to me on many accounts; but it must be remember'd that Mr. Gervis's Letters giving an account of the Ashburton Case[2] were in the hands of Mr. Aikin[3] several weeks, & I was in hopes he would have moulded them into form. I should then have furnish'd him with Mrs. Wake's Letter.[4] Another fact of a similar nature to Mrs. Wake's which took place in a noble family, I find myself not at liberty to publish. However I have put what matter I possess'd into as good a form as I could, and as it so strongly supports a theory I have long maintain'd, you will see by the printed Paper accompanying this,[5] in what manner I have managed it. Observe, this Paper is not publish'd, nor intended to be publish'd; at least till the *Verulam* Socy.[6] have made what use they please of it. They may print the whole if they please, or the Cases at the latter end only,[7] with the introduction I have already written & placed in the hands of Mr. Aikin.

The Paper on *the Distemper* among Dogs,[8] I hope to make more complete than it is at present in the course of a short space of time but yet I fear not time enough for the first number of the Societies Communications. I wait to dissect some Dogs that are not diseas'd,[9] as I am not certain, whether an appearance that presents itself in the diseas'd Dogs on the Dura Mater, is a natural Plexus of Vessels, or inflammation. Moseley could *tell me no doubt,* but I don't like to ask favors of him.[10]

Believe me with sincere regards, & best wishes to you & yours in which Mrs. Jenner joins me,

Your faithful Friend & Servant

E. Jenner

PS. Poor Knowles I hear is praying heartily to be reinstated in his situation at the Central House.[11] His late embarrassment appears to have arisen more from misfortune than criminality. He lent money & could not get paid again, & this sent him into temporary durance. I understand out of his slender income, he has nearly maintain'd two little sisters who were destitute. Let this meritorious act plead for him.

---

1. See Letter 7, n. 1.

2. Henry Gervis, a surgeon at Ashburton in Devonshire, had written Jenner of a woman vaccinated during the last month of pregnancy who gave birth to a baby infected with smallpox.

3. Charles Rochemont Aikin (1775–1847) was secretary of the Medical and Chirurgical Society.

4. Mrs. Wake was the mother of an infant which, when vaccinated, was immune to cowpox. It was learned that a few days before her confinement, she had met a man ill with

smallpox. Although Mrs. Wake was immune, having had smallpox as a child, her baby developed a few smallpox pustules, from which it recovered, shortly after its birth.

5. Jenner is referring to the pamphlet *Facts, for the most part unobserved, or not duly noticed, respecting Variolous Contagion* (London: Printed by S. Gosnell, 1808) (LeFanu 85), evidently in a printed form prior to publication. This contains a description of the two cases mentioned above.

6. The Medical and Chirurgical Society met at 2, Verulam Buildings, Gray's Inn.

7. On 4 April 1809 Jenner read a paper to the Medical and Chirurgical Society on "Two cases of small-pox infection communicated to the foetus in utero under peculiar circumstances, with additional remarks," excerpted from the paper cited in n. 5, above. This was published in *Medico-Chirurgical Transactions* 1 (1809): 269–75 (LeFanu 90). See also Letter 39.

8. Read to the Medical and Chirurgical Society on 21 March 1809 and published in *Medico-Chirurgical Transactions* 1 (1809): 263–68 (LeFanu 87). Jenner evidently began his studies on the distemper in dogs in 1796. The notebook of Edward Jenner in the possession of the Royal College of Physicians of London (published with an introduction by F. Dawtrey Drewitt, London, 1931 [LeFanu 121]) contains observations on dissections of dead dogs in 1796, 1804, and 1806.

9. It is doubtful that Jenner performed these dissections, since his published paper does not mention it. For further details see Letter 39.

10. See Letter 18, n. 4. Moseley had published *On Hydrophobia, its Prevention and Cure. With a description of the different stages of canine madness: illustrated with cases* (London, 1808).

11. James Sheridan Knowles (see Letter 34, n. 2), resident vaccinator of the Jennerian Society at the Central House in Salisbury Square, failed to inspire confidence among his patients. He later became a distinguished playwright and actor, but his artistic temperament was little appreciated by his medical colleagues. James Moore in his *History and Practice of Vaccination* (London, 1817) writes of him: "The new Vaccinator was jocund and volatile, and fancied himself a poet; though his faint inspirations were only produced by the bewitching juice of the little western flower called love in idleness. He hated the trammels of business, and always had a ready gibe to flout at order. So, when mothers brought their children early in the morning to be vaccinated, he was sometimes fast asleep; and when they carried them late, he had perhaps strolled abroad. Even when seated seriously at home, the drudgery of registering cases was apt to be postponed, while he was listlessly rhyming a piteous sonnet to his sempstress. Such a character was far from irreclaimable; but the Vaccine might have languished long, and the Small Pox might have made wasteful havoc, before the boiling spirits of this juvenile Hibernian could be cooled down to the medical point" (p. 216).

38. To Dr. Thomas Charles Morgan, Peterhouse, Cambridge, 20 December 1808

My dear Doctor [1]

There is nothing enlivens a Cottage Fireside, remote from the Capital, so much as a Newspaper. The Pilot of last night was particularly cheering, as it told me you had finish'd your academic labors & received your Honors.

Allow me to congratulate you, & to assure you how happy I shall ever be in hearing of anything that adds to your Fame, your fortune; or to your general comforts. [*Three lines crossed out.*] The horrid Fever my eldest Son has undergone has left him quite a Wreck;[2] but I don't despair of seeing him restored. I should be quite at ease on the subject, if a little Cough did not still hang upon him, & too quick a pulse.

The Regius Professor of Phys: in the university of Cambridge corresponding with the contemptible Editors of that miserable Catchpenny Journal, the Medical Observer!!![3] What Phaenomenon, I wonder, will Vaccination next present to us? Atrocious & absurd as this man's conduct has been, there will be a difficulty in punishing him, as he seems insensible to everything but his own Conceit. However he is in able hands, and my excellent Friend Thackary[4] (to whom I beg you to remember me most kindly) I know will not spare him. Sr. Isaac has certainly out blockheaded all his Predecessors. Pray tell me what is going forward. Alas! poor Ring![5] He has been too daring, & I tremble for his fate. The Scourge[6] is out, and I don't see that he erased a single line that was pointed out to him as dangerous. This venemous sting will produce a most troublesome reaction, & injure the cause it was meant to support. You know the pains I took to suppress it; but all would not do.

I have not heard anything of the new Vaccine Institution since my arrival here, except a word or two from Lord Egremont,[7] who says the Ministry are so incessantly occupied with the affairs of Spain,[8] that matters of a minor consideration cannot at present be attended to. I shall thank my Friend in Russell Square,[9] for the communications which, thro' you, he was good enough to make to me, but am of opinion that the proper time to object, will be when anything objectionable rises up. Whatever is going forward either in the College or out of it, is at present carefully conceal'd from me. The proposition hinted at by Dr. S.[10] respecting an equal number from both Colleges to form the Board, I mention'd to Sr. Lucas[11] as the certain means of keeping off those jealousies, which otherwise I thought would shew themselves. It affords me great pleasure to assure you that your Pamphlet[12] is *much* liked by all who have read it, in this part of the World and by no one more than by myself. A few trifling alterations will be necessary for the *next Edition.* I think you may be more copious in your extracts from some of those Letters of which Murray avail'd himself. By the bye, it might not be amiss perhaps if, by way of firing a Shot at the head of your Knight,[13] the extract from Sacco's[14] Letter (see Murray's Appendix)[15] & that from Dr. Keir[16] at Bombay, were to appear in the Cambridge Newspaper.

With the best wishes of myself and Family, believe me, Dear Doctor
Most faithfully   Yours

Edw. Jenner

Berkeley
Decr. 20 1808

1. Dr. (later Sir) Thomas Charles Morgan (1783–1843), who a few years later married Sydney Owenson, a popular Irish authoress. At this time he had just received his M.D. degree from Cambridge, from whence he had graduated M.B. in 1804. This letter is published in full in *Lady Morgan's Memoirs: Autobiography, Diaries, and Correspondence* (London, 1862), 1:374–76. See also Letters 40, 46, 49, and 51.

2. Jenner's son Edward had recovered from typhus. He died in February 1810 from pulmonary tuberculosis. See Letters 46, 49, 51, and 53.

3. Sir Isaac Pennington (1745–1817) had sent a report to the Royal College of Physicians of twenty-five cases of smallpox in Cambridge which occurred among people who had previously been vaccinated. The editor of the *Medical Observer* wrote to ask Pennington's opinion of the cases, and the correspondence was printed in the *Medical Observer*, 4 (December 1808): 240–48. The *Medical Observer; or, Monthly Expositor of regular and irregular Quackery* was a popular journal that began publication in 1806. One of its chief purposes was to combat vaccination.

4. Frederic Thackeray, a surgeon at Cambridge, had defended vaccination in the face of Sir Isaac Pennington's unfavorable report by publishing a letter in the *Cambridge Chronicle* on 5 November 1808. This letter is reprinted in the *Medical Observer* 4 (December 1808): 241–43.

5. John Ring. See Letter 33.

6. [John Ring], *The Vaccine Scourge, in answer to the calumnies and falsehoods, lately circulated with great industry by that extraordinary surgeon, Mr. Birch, and other anti-vaccinists* (London: J. Murray, 1808). It contained a long poem with explanatory notes ridiculing the opponents of vaccination.

7. Plans were under way to establish a new vaccine institution under governmental auspices to replace the nearly defunct Jennerian Society. Lord Egremont was Sir George O'Brien Wyndham (1751–1837).

8. The Peninsular War against Napoleon was going on at this time.

9. Dr. Alexander Marcet was now living on Russell Square.

10. William Saunders, M.D. (1743–1817), a prominent London physician.

11. Sir Lucas Pepys (1742–1830), president of the Royal College of Physicians of London. The board met for the first time a week after this letter was written, on 28 December 1808. It was composed of the president and censors of the College of Physicians and the master and governors of the College of Surgeons of London.   — James Moore, *The History and Practice of Vaccination* (London, 1817), p. 222.

12. Probably Morgan's *An Expostulatory Letter to Dr. Moseley, on his Review of the Report of the London College of Physicians on Vaccination* (London, 1808).

13. Sir Isaac Pennington.

14. Luigi Sacco (1769–1836) was the chief exponent of vaccination in Italy. Beginning in September 1800, when he first became acquainted with Jenner's discovery, he fought actively against smallpox, was named director of vaccination in Lombardy, and published several books on his experiences.

15. Charles Murray, *An answer to Mr. Highmore's objections to the Bill before Parliament to prevent*

the spreading of the small pox; with an appendix containing some interesting communications from foreign medical practitioners, on the progress and efficacy of vaccine inoculation (London, 1808).

16. George Keir had performed early vaccinations in India, beginning in June 1802. His *Account of the introduction of the cow-pox into India* was published in Bombay in 1803. See *de Carro–Marcet Letters,* p. 59.

39. To Dr. Alexander J. G. Marcet, Russell Square, London, 17 January 1809

My dear Sir[1]

I never had a more earnest desire to fulfil an engagement than that I made with you respecting the Paper on the Distemper among Dogs;[2] but such have been my incessant occupations since my arrival here, that I have had no time to bestow on anything not immediately professional, or what was connected with the business of the National Vaccine Institution,[3] which I may say to you is by no means fashion'd to my liking, but on the contrary, arranged very awkwardly. You will hear more of this.

I will explain what seems to puzzle you respecting the printed Paper "Facts respecting variolous contagion &c."[4] It was my intention to have given the Society the Cases only which appear at the end of the Paper, to shew the fact that in the advanc'd state of pregnancy, a female may, by exposure to variolous contagion communicate the smallpox to the Foetus altho' she herself has previously gone thro' the disease. This of course required introductory remarks, & these I had drawn up & shew'd to Mr. Aikin one day when he call'd upon me in Russell Street. If you print the whole Paper, these, of course, will not be wanted. Two Copies only, to the best of my recollection, were dispos'd of; the rest are secured, & shall remain so till your Volume comes out.

If the Press is still open, & you still think your first Work too small, I will do the best I can with the Paper on the Dog distemper & send it to you — It may do pretty well with some such Title as this "Cursory Observations &c."[5]

Believe me   my dear Sir   most truly Yours

Edw. Jenner

Berkeley
Jan: 17 1809

I expect to be in Town early in the ensuing Month.

1. For the other Marcet letters, see Letter 7, n. 1.
2. See Letter 37. Marcet was evidently begging Jenner to send in his paper "Distemper among Dogs" for publication in the *Medico-Chirurgical Transactions.*

3. See Letters 38 and 40. When the National Vaccine Establishment was created, Jenner was appointed director; however, when he began to appoint the vaccinators, most of his nominees were rejected by the board. A letter of 9 January 1809 from Jenner to his close friend Thomas Pruen preserved at the Wellcome Historical Medical Library gives the following information: "The affairs of the National Vaccine Establishment go on badly. I am got into the *cleft stick* completely, as you shall hear. The Board appointed me Director of course, but they have contriv'd to let me know that I am the Director directed; for out of the eight names I nominated to fill the Vaccinating Stations, they have taken only two; the others are fill'd by men who are utter strangers to me, and what is still worse (indeed is it not insulting?) one of them who is appointed the Vaccine Chief, & to superintend the other Stations, is really taken from Pearson's Institution [Vaccine Pock Institution in Golden Square; see Letter 17, n. 2], to which he was surgeon. [*Crossed out*] Keate, the very man who link'd himself with Pearson to form his Institution, & the very man who made a base attempt to upset me in the Committee of the House of Commons, is one of the Board. The question is then, shall I immediately resign & shew them a little of the indignation I feel, or wait till I have cooly taken the opinion of my Friends? At all events as I observ'd, I must be embroil'd, and this is the more calamitous, as it happens at the very time when I hoped for some domestic repose, after ten years hard & incessant labor. By submission, what am I but an underling in an Institution in which Pearson will, thro' his agents virtually take the lead; and to resist & thereby gain my point, will throw me upon a bed of Vipers; for not only those who by a struggle on my part may be dismiss'd, but their numerous adherents, will be forever wounding me with their Fangs. I may most piteously exclaim, what shall I do?" Jenner did resign as director. See Baron, *Life,* 2:120–31.

4. See Letter 37 for details about this publication.

5. The published title was "Observations on the Distemper in Dogs" (LeFanu 87).

40. To Dr. Thomas Charles Morgan, 109 Great Russell St., Bedford Square, London, 1 March 1809

My dear Sir[1]

I ought to make a thousand apologies to you for suffering your last obliging Letter to remain so long unanswer'd. Did my Friends whom I serve in this manner, but know the worrying kind of life I lead, they would soon seal my pardon. However I feel myself now more at ease than for some time past, having crept from under the *thick, heavy* Board,[2] which so unexpectedly fell upon me & crush'd me so sorely. To speak more plainly, I have inform'd the Gentlemen in Leicester Square, that I cannot accept of the office to which they nominated me. Should the business come before the Public, as I suppose it will, I am not afraid of an honorable acquittal. Never was anything so clumsily managed. If Sr. Isaac[3] himself, instead of Sr. Lucas,[4] had taken the lead, it could not have been worse, as I shall convince you when we come to talk the matter over. By the way, what is become of this right valiant Knight?[5] Thackeray, I hope, has not done exchanging Lances with him, unless he is ashamed of the Contest. I was glad to see your Pamphlet advertis'd on the *yellow Cover*. Give it as much publicity as you please, & remember you are to draw on me for all Costs. Does it go off, or sleep with the pages of Moseley? [6] Opposition to Vaccination seems dead — at least in this part of the World we hear nothing of it. Thro' a vast District around me, I don't know a man who ever unsheaths that most venomous of all Weapons, the Variolous Lancet. [7] And the Smallpox, if it now & then seizes upon some deluded Infidel, soon dies away for want of more prey. I have not written to my Friend Dr. Saunders [8] a long time, but if you see him, assure him he shall hear soon from me. If he considers the business between me & the Board, & looks steadfastly on all its bearings, I am confident he will not condemn my Conduct. If it should be thought of consequence enough for an Enquiry, I shall meet it with pleasure; but tho' I say "with pleasure," I had much rather they would let me alone, and suffer me to smoke my Seagar in peace & quietness in my Cottage.

My Boys are better — How is your little Cherub? Adieu, my dear Sir — Most truly Yours

Edw. Jenner

Berkeley
March 1st 1809

1. See Letter 38.

2. Jenner is referring to the board of the newly created National Vaccine Establishment in Leicester Square, of which he had been named director. See Letter 39.

3. Sir Isaac Pennington, whose antivaccination activities are discussed in Jenner's previous letter to Morgan, Letter 38.

4. Sir Lucas Pepys, president of the Royal College of Physicians of London and a member of the board of the National Vaccine Establishment.

5. Sir Isaac.

6. Morgan's pamphlet was directed against the antivaccinist Moseley. See Letter 38, n. 12.

7. Smallpox inoculation, or variolation.

8. See Letter 38, n. 10. Saunders was the first president of the Medical and Chirurgical Society.

41. To Dr. Alexander J. G. Marcet, Russell Square, London, 12 March 1809

Berkeley
March 12 1809

My dear Sir [1]

The object I had in view in throwing together these remarks, was to elucidate the laws of Physiology concerning such infections as the Variolous

& Vaccine. For this purpose, I deem'd it expedient to reprint the observations which I publish'd ten years ago, lest my enforcing those doctrines at present by new evidence should be spoken of as a subterfuge to screen the reputed failures of Vaccination. The fresh Facts, relating to the infection of the Foetus by Mothers who had previously had the Smallpox or Cowpox, I adduce as striking illustrations of my opinion. I therefore conceive that one part of the little Treatise in your hands, depends upon the other, and that they cannot well be separated. If, however, it be more agreeable to you and the Council to introduce into their volume the Foetus Cases only, I shall have no objection, and have therefore enclos'd some remarks that may serve as an introduction to the Paper.[2]

The Paper on the Dog-distemper still remains unarranged. If possible, I will send it you in time.[3] If I do not, you must attribute it to that embarrassment which absolute necessity has driven me into. It was not without extreme regret, that I withdrew myself from the National Vaccine Establishment;[4] but after what had happen'd, I found my Post untenable, consistently with the duty I owed my Country, my Friends & myself.

Believe me   ever most faithfully Yours

Edw. Jenner

Pray present mine & Mrs. Jenner's best regards to Mrs. Marcet.

1. For the other Marcet letters, see Letter 7, n. 1.
2. The paper was finally published in the form suggested here, with only the fetus cases included, in *Medico-Chirurgical Transactions* 1 (1809): 269–75. For previous discussions of this paper see Letters 37 and 39.
3. This was published in the same volume of the *Medico-Chirurgical Transactions* as the paper on fetuses (1:263–65). See also Letters 37, 39, and 42.
4. See Letter 39, n. 3.

42.   To Dr. Alexander J. G. Marcet, 15 March 1809

My dear Doctr.[1]

In the midst of my new embarrassment, I have stol'n time enough to arrange the *Dog Paper,*[2] & you shall have it by Monday's Post.

I hope my Friends in Town will contradict a rumour, wherever they find it, (& it is put about with considerable industry) that I seceded from the new Institution,[3] because its whole management was not put into my hands. Nothing was ever further from my thoughts or wishes. My reputation, when the motives that guided my conduct come to be publicly known, I trust will suffer no stain; but there would have been an indelible blot upon it, had I acted otherwise; at least such is my opinion.

Have you seen Professor Sr. Munck Rosenschold from Sweden?[4] He has paid me a visit and brings with him one of the grandest Reports of Vaccination, that has yet been presented to me. If I understood him right (for he speaks english imperfectly, & I nothing but my Mother Tongue) he has been enobled[5] on account of his gigantic & successful efforts, in banishing the smallpox from the Swedish Dominions.

Our kindest regards to Mrs. Marcet.

Truly Yours

E Jenner

15 March 1809

1. For the other Marcet letters, see Letter 7, n. 1.

2. See preceding Letter 41.

3. The National Vaccine Establishment, of which Jenner had been appointed the first director and then resigned. See Letter 39, n. 3.

4. Eberhard Zacharias Munck af Rosenschöld (1775–1837) introduced vaccination into Sweden. He first learned about vaccination in May 1801, when he was in Copenhagen. The following October he began vaccinating in Skaane, the southwestern province of Sweden, with lymph which he procured in Copenhagen. By the end of 1801 he had vaccinated 2,000 in Skaane, and from there he sent material to the other provinces, sparing no pains in writing or making trips to promote vaccination in Sweden. For his work he was elected to membership and awarded a medal by the Kongl. Patriotiska Sällskapet (Royal Patriotic Society). —Joh. Fredr. Sacklén, *Sveriges Läkare-Historia* (Nyköping, 1822), pp. 666–71.

5. Jenner misunderstood him. Munck af Rosenschöld was raised to the nobility, together with the other members of his family, in 1799, before he had had anything to do with vaccination.

43. To Dr. Alexander J. G. Marcet, Russell Square, London, 26 March 1809

My dear Sir[1]

I am a little impatient to know what you intend doing with my Papers.[2] Will you have the goodness just to write a line or two & tell me?

I have religiously kept my promise in not circulating the printed Paper,[3] altho' I want to do it exceedingly, for reasons that must be obvious.

Is there a possibility of getting Letters into Holland or Germany? Some have lately reach'd me from Berlin and Rotterdam, which I much wish to answer. King Louis[4] I find is a very warm promoter of Vaccination in his dominions.

Believe me   truly Yours

E Jenner

Berkeley
26 March 1809

1. For the other Marcet letters, see Letter 7, n. 1.

2. See Letters 37, 39, 41, and 42.

3. The pamphlet *Facts, for the most part unobserved, or not duly noticed, respecting Variolous Contagion* (London: printed by S. Gosnell, 1808) (LeFanu 85). The cases described therein were also being published in the *Medico-Chirurgical Transactions*.

4. Louis Bonaparte, Napoleon's third brother, had been made king of Holland in 1806.

44. To William Blair, Esq., Great Russell St., Bloomsbury, London, 26 April 1809

Berkeley Apl. 26 1809

My dear Sir[1]

Out of delicacy to some of the Members who constitute the Board of the National Vaccine Establishment, for there are among them respectable Men, I took the liberty of requesting you, as well as some other Friends of mine in Town, not to be in a hurry in bringing forward any public observations. I don't know that such a restriction is necessary now, for really a total silence on the subject may be injurious to my reputation. I know it has been industriously said, that my secession arose from disappointment in not being allow'd to have the sole management of the Institution in my own hands.[2] Nothing can be further from the Truth. I never had, or ever intimated, such a wish. All I wanted was the appointment of such Persons to the vaccinating Department, as from my own knowledge, were intimately acquainted with the practice and for whom I could be responsible.[3] But you know how this business was managed; & how I was insulted (was it not an insult?) by their selecting one, & appointing him the *Chief,* from an Institution that had always most wantonly opposed me & my doctrines. Yet perhaps you may not know that the New Institution is form'd for the purpose of investigating the merits of the vaccine practice, and that from this Enquiry the public are to know whether it be really beneficial or dangerous.[4] And this forsooth comes out as the reason why I could not possibly be one of the Board, as the public would not then have been so well satisfied with the decision. This would have been very well some years ago, but now it is an insult to common sense. I am astonish'd how the College, after their late Report, could take upon themselves an office so degrading! Is it possible the "auri sacra fames" can have so beguil'd their senses, or what can be their motive? To say nothing of the long & solemn Trial of Vaccination in Warwick Lane,[5] has it not been at the Bar, the great Tribunal of the world, & loudly pronounc'd to be what my Investigations warranted me to proclaim it, safe & efficacious? The Colleges in thus inadvertently degrading me, will undoubtedly injure themselves. But, my good Sir, notwithstanding all that has hitherto happen'd, I think it would be most prudent for me at present to remain silent. From intimations I have received, there is little doubt that an Inquiry will be made in an august assembly as to the disposal of the money granted for the support of the Establishment. The whole business will then be developed, and that will be the moment for me to go into an explanation of my conduct. As to the common voice of defamation, which in the meantime may attempt to annoy me, I shall treat it with contempt. I have written to Addington,[6] in answer to an Inquiry of his, respecting the R. J. Socy.[7] —

Mrs. Jenner begs me to thank you for your Communications, but wishes they had been more pleasant.

Remember me kindly to my Friend Rich'd Phillips[8] when you see him, & talk this affair over with him. It is very uncertain when I may come to Town — I hope not this Spring. Remember I spent seven months there lately, doing no manner of good to the public & an immense injury to myself & Family. Good accounts of Vaccination pour in upon me from all quarters. The *only* Child of a Family of distinction in this County is just dead under Smallpox Inoculation.

Believe me truly Yours

Edw: Jenner

PS.   Should not Mr. Wilberforce[9] be made acquainted with the Conduct of *the Board*? I don't think it would be so prudent for me to make the Communication as some other person. I never have been able to obtain a sight of the Secretary of State's Warrant to the College.[10] How could I get a sight of it?

1. William Blair (1766–1822), surgeon, had been director of the Royal Jennerian Society. For his publications supporting vaccination see Letter 33, n. 9. See also Letter 45.

2. For details see Letter 39, n. 3.

3. Jenner had nominated his friend John Ring as principal vaccinator and inspector of stations. Instead, the board appointed J. C. Carpue (1764–1846), a disciple of Dr. George Pearson, who had earlier attacked Jenner (see Letter 8, n. 3 and Letter 17, n. 2).

4. For an elaboration of this point, see a letter Jenner wrote on 4 April 1809 to his friend James Moore in Baron, *Life*, 2:126–28.

5. The Royal College of Physicians of London was situated on Warwick Lane.

6. John Addington. See Letter 12.

7. The Royal Jennerian Society. See Letter 12, n. 4.

8. See Letter 20.

9. William Wilberforce (1759–1833), the philanthropist and crusader against slavery, was

a member of Parliament who had ardently supported the founding of the National Vaccine Establishment.

10. The warrant for instituting the National Vaccine Establishment had been sent to Sir Lucas Pepys, president of the College of Physicians, by Lord Hawkesbury, the secretary of state for the Home Department.

45. To William Blair, Esq., Great Russell St., Bloomsbury, London, 9 June 1809

Berkeley   June 9 1809

My dear Sir[1]

I am making up a Packet of Letters for my Friends in Town to go by one of my Neighbours. You must not be forgotten, tho' you are a Letter in my debt.

My Conduct respecting the new Institution,[2] I find has drawn down upon me some severe censures; but as nothing reaches me but in vague, untangible shape, I cannot make any reply. The Letter to Mr. J. Moore in the last Med: Observer[3] seems from the style to come from Moseley.[4] We shall see whether Moore will notice it — I should suppose, he will not.

I am happy to see this vile Publication (the Observer) so well taken to task by the Med: Spectator.[5] We sometimes find Friends in places where we little expect to see them. Who my Friend & Defender is, I know not, perhaps you can tell me, & will have the goodness to do it. I certainly feel obliged to him. Sr. Rich'd Phillips[6] call'd on me a few days ago & inform'd me that not more than 250 of the Observers were now printed. These can do but little harm. Will the Spectator rise as this sinks? I express'd myself in strong terms to Sr. Richard respecting the line of conduct now pursued in the Med: & Phys: Journal. He said as much of Dr. A — —[7] in reply as accounted for the change. Bradley, he said, he did not see once in three months. *A — — has strongly urged the Knight & his Lady to have their Children variolated! — This tender solicitation of the Doctor's, was accompanied with such remarks on Vaccination as I should have thought would better have harmoniz'd with the Tongue of Moseley!* — At present, don't say anything of this communication, except in confidence.

In haste   truly Yours

Edw. Jenner

PS.   The R. J. Socy.[8] I hear is still in being, & that efforts will be made to give it fresh vigour. I certainly shall not be backward in lending my aid; but all my Friends must see the delicate situation in which it places me; as I by no means think the Nat: Vac: Establishment will remain long in its present state of organization. I hope my Friend Addington[9] has long since produc'd my Letter on this Subject, at one of your Meetings.

P.S.   Mrs. Jenner begs to be kindly remember'd to you.
Will you have the kindness to inform me who the important Mr. Davis[10] is, that assails you in the Med: Journal?

1. See Letter 44.
2. The National Vaccine Establishment. See the preceding letter.
3. *The Medical Observer, and Family Monitor* 6 (June 1809): 78–80. The letter was addressed "To Mr. Moore, Assistant-Director of the National Vaccine Establishment" and signed "Chirurgus." The author commented upon the difficulty of Moore's position as a result of Jenner's secession from the Establishment, for now Moore must be the defender both of the "errors of vaccination" and the conduct of its discoverer. The recent cases of smallpox at Cheltenham, "the grand theatre of Dr. Jenner's experiments," were mentioned. The published "Instructions respecting Vaccination" issued by the National Vaccine Establishment were also criticized.
4. Benjamin Moseley, M.D., Jenner's archenemy. See Letter 18, n. 5.
5. *London Medical and Surgical Spectator; or, Monthly Register of Medicine in Its Various Branches.* Only two volumes appeared, in 1808 and 1809.
6. See Letter 20. Phillips is also mentioned in Letter 44.
7. Dr. Joseph Adams (1756–1818) was editor of the *Medical and Physical Journal,* together with Dr. T. Bradley.
8. The Royal Jennerian Society. See Letter 12, n. 4.
9. John Addington. See Letter 12.
10. In the *Medical and Physical Journal* 21 (1809): 121–25, a Mr. J. Davies had criticized the Jennerian Society, asserting that its members were deaf to evidence contrary to their convictions. William Blair, in a brief letter in reply (ibid., p. 438), inquired if he were included in the censure and wanted to know on what grounds the letter-writer "ventures to insinuate such a charge of obliquity in my moral and medical character," and whether Davies had read his publications. Davies retorted (pp. 478–80) that Blair's prejudice would never permit him to see the truth, and that he (Davies) never intended to read Blair's publications.

46.   To Dr. Thomas Charles Morgan, Great Russell St., Bedford Square, London, 11 July 1809

My dear Sir[1]
You have some heavy accusations I know to bring against me on the subject of my long silence. I have no other excuse to offer you than that of pecuniary Bankrupts, who have so many debts, that they discharge none. However deficient I may have been in writing, I have not been so in thinking of you & your kind attentions. If you have seen your Neighbour Blair[2] lately, he must have told you so.

You supposed me at Cheltenham when you wrote last. Unfortunately I have not yet been able to quit this place, and have been detain'd by a sad business, the still existing illness of my eldest Son,[3] the young Man who was so ill when I was in Town. His appearance for some time past, flatter'd me with a hope that he was convalescent, but to my great affliction he was seiz'd Saturday last with Haemorrhage from the Lungs, which return'd yesterday & today exactly at the same hour, almost at the same minute; seven in the morning. This is a melancholy prospect for me, & I scarcely know how to bear it. The decrees of Heaven, however harsh they may seem, must be correct, & the grand Lesson we have to learn is humility.

I wrote two long argumentative Letters to Dr. Saunders[4] soon after I rec'd your hint, on the subject of the new Institution;[5] but from that time he has dropp'd his correspondence with me. When next you fall in with the Doctor, pray sound him on this subject. Have you seen the last number of that infamous Publication, the Medl. Observer? There is the most impudent Letter in it from the Editor to me, that ever was penn'd.[6] I think our Friend Harry would at once pronounce it grossly libellous. The thing I am abused for, the effects of an epidemic Smallpox at Cheltenham, is as triumphant as any that has occur'd in the annals of Vaccin'n. A Child that had irregular Pustules, & was on that account order'd by me to be revaccinated, which order was never obey'd, caught the Smallpox. This is the whole of the matter & on this foundation Moseley, Birch[7] & Co. have heap'd up a mountain of scurrility. Between 3 & 4000 persons have been vaccinated there & in the circumjacent Villages *who remain'd in the midst of the Epidemic* untouch'd. This *trifling* circumstance these worthy Gentlemen did not think worth their while to mention. Adieu my dear Sir — I hope you are very well & very happy.

Most truly Yours

E. Jenner

Berkeley   11 July 1809

---

1. See Letters 38, 40, 49, and 51.

2. Both Morgan and William Blair (Letters 44 and 45) lived on Great Russell St.

3. Edward Jenner, Jr., who died from pulmonary tuberculosis in February 1810. See also Letters 38, 49, and 51.

4. Dr. William Saunders, mentioned in Letters 38 and 40.

5. The National Vaccine Establishment.

6. In *The Medical Observer, and Family Monitor* 6 (July 1809): 86–90, the editor pointed to the cases of smallpox which developed at Cheltenham early that year as evidence that vaccination is worthless. A letter from Mr. Freeman, surgeon and apothecary of Cheltenham, was reprinted. It described five cases of smallpox among children who had been vaccinated four or five years previously, four of them by Jenner himself.

7. See Letter 19, n. 7.

47. To T. Cobb, Esq., Banbury, Oxfordshire, 8 August 1809

Berkeley Glostre.

August 8 1809

Dear Sir[1]

Your Letter has just reach'd me at Berkeley. I have been prevented from going to Cheltenham at my usual time from the severe indisposition of my eldest Son, whose health is still in a very alarming state.[2]

I am sorry to hear that Mrs. Cobb is so unwell. Pray assure her I should be happy to suggest any medicinal plan for the restoration of her health. Faintings, such as you describe, are not very uncommon in Constitutions dispos'd to be hysterical. Has Mr. Hayward,[3] or have you perceived any Symptom of this malady in Mrs. Cobb? Such as a sense of a Ball's rising in the Gullet & affecting the Breath — making suddenly a quantity of pale Urine, irregular Spirits &c &c. Or has Mr. H. any suspicion that the pain preceeding the Fainting arose from Gall Stones? I throw out these questions as hints for enquiry. However be the cause what it may, some mild Tonics will probably be beneficial and with these I should unite tepid Bathing three or four times a week at a temperature of 95. The time for using the Bath for those who are debilitated I have commonly found to be most agreeable about midway between breakfast & dinner — she might remain in it from fifteen to thirty or forty minutes, indeed as long as it is pleasant to her feelings. — It would also be certainly advisable for her to keep her bowels constantly open by means of some very mild aperient. A large Teaspoonful of Epsom Salts dissolv'd in a full half-pint of warm Water may be taken daily before breakfast, like Cheltenham Water — the quantity may be increas'd or diminish'd according to its effects. It is not intended to act as a direct purgative, but only to give one, or at most two evacuations daily.

Enclos'd is a Prescription for a tonic Medicine, which I think will answer a good purpose, as she cannot bear the Bark.[4] Mrs. Jenner begs her best Comps. With best wishes to you and Mrs. Cobb, I remain

Dear Sir   Truly Yours

Edw. Jenner

PS.   Your Letter, tho' single was charged double — I should not have noticed this to you, had it not appear'd to me to have been open'd before it reach'd my hands. How is my old Friend Shorter?

[*Attached prescription:*][5]

Rp Quassiae ʒ i
    Aquae Ferventis pt ss
Macera per horam et cola.

Rp Liquoris Colat: ℥ vii
 Magnesiae ℈ iv
 Zinci Vitriolat: praep: gr ii
 T. Cardam: Comp: ℥ i M[isce].
Sumat Cocli: iii ampla meridie et vespere.

Mrs. Cobb
 Augusti 8vo
  1809   E J.

 1. See Letters 13 and 48.
 2. See Letter 46, n. 3.
 3. The family surgeon, who has not been identified.
 4. Peruvian bark, or cinchona.
 5. I am indebted to Dr. Owsei Temkin and Dr. G. R. Paterson for assisting in transcribing and translating this prescription. It reads:

> "Take 1 dram of Quassia, ½ pt. of hot water, soak for an hour and strain. Take 7 ounces of the strained liquid, 4 scruples of magnesia, 2 grains of zinc sulphate, and 1 ounce of compound tincture of cardamom. Mix. Take 3 ample spoonfuls at noon and in the evening.
> Mrs. Cobb
> August 8, 1809   E. J."

48. To T. Cobb, Esq., [before September 1815]

Dr. Jenner's Comps. to Mr. Cobb[1] — He would advise him to take the Cheltenham Waters regularly during his stay here without the interference of any other Medicine. He would wish him to take three second-siz'd Glasses to morrow morning & to desire Mrs. Forty to give it of the degree of heat Dr. J. recommends.

The imperfection in the first made Pills is now too palpable to admit of further doubt.

Tuesday Evening [Cheltenham][2]

[Undated fragment]
The long continued use of a tepid Bath. The temperature at first may be 92 degrees of the Thermometer, & it may gradually be reduc'd to 82 if Mr. Cobb's feelings will admit.

Some mild aperient to prevent costiveness — Either the Pill Mr. Cobb has spoken of, or the Cheltenham Salts dissolv'd in water, so as to imitate that at the Spa.

If the pain in the head should continue, let Blisters be applied in succession near the seat of it, & use twice a day a pinch of Cephalic Snuff. The *Pulvis Assari Composit:* (to be procured at No. 136 New Bond St.) will answer the purpose very well. Circumspection with respect to diet, Mr. C. will find to be a very important consideration.

1. See Letters 13 and 47.

2. The letter bears an orange seal, which indicates that it was written before Mrs. Jenner died in September 1815; thereafter the seal was black. This letter has been placed here because of the similarity of its content to the previous letter, also addressed to Cobb.

49. To Dr. Thomas Charles Morgan, Ramsgate, Kent, 9 October 1809

My dear Sir[1]

You may easily guess what a state of mind I am in, by my neglecting my Friends. This I was not wont to do. I am grown as moping as the Owl, and all the day long sit brooding over Melancholy. My poor Boy still exists, but is wasting inch by inch. The ray of Hope is denied only to a medical Man when he sees his Child dying of pulmonary Consumption; all other Mortals enjoy its flattering light. You say nothing of your little Girl in your Letter from Ramsgate — I hope she is well & will prove a lasting Comfort to you.

If Dr. Saunders[2] is displeas'd, his displeasure can have no other grounds than caprice. I never did anything in my life that should have call'd it up. I wrote twice to him in the Spring, & since that time he has not written to me. Why, I am utterly at a loss to know. In one of these Letters I went fully into an explanation of my conduct with regard to the National Vac: Estabt.[3] — Depend upon it neither Mr. R[4] nor Sr. Lucas will ever make it the subject of public Enquiry. They know better. I have always treated the College with due respect. They made an admirable Report to Parliament of Vaccination;[5] but in doing this they shew'd me no favor. It was founded on the general evidence sent in from every part of the Empire. I love to feel sensible of an obligation, where it is due, & to shew my gratitude. If the College had publish'd the Evidence, which they promis'd to do, then I should have been greatly obligated to them. Why this was not done, I never could learn, but shall ever lament that such valuable facts should lie mouldering on their Shelves, as they must from their weight have lain too heavy on the Tongue of Clamour for it ever to have moved again. I wish you had been there, & that I had first made my acquaintance with you. One strenuous Friend in Warwick Lane[6] would have effected every thing, by filling up this lamentable Chasm.

I enjoy'd your Dialogue. *Poor* Sr. Isaac![7] Your Pamphlet[8] is highly spoken of, wherever it is read — after this *Spree* of your Talents in lashing the Antivaccinists, I hope you don't mean to lay down the Rod. Moseley, as far as I have seen, has not taken the least notice of it, a proof of his Tremors; for he has not been sparing of his other Opponents. And now my good Friend let me request you without delay to let me know the expences of printing, advertisements &c &c &c. I don't exactly know where this may find you, but shall get a Cover[9] for Ramsgate — If you are not there it will pursue you. Dr. Saunders's throwing me off, I assure you vexes me; but I have the consolation of knowing that it was unmerited.

Remember me kindly to our Friend *Harry*. He will soon climb the Hill I think — He may be assured of not reaching the top a day sooner than I wish him. Will you have the goodness when in Town to order Harwood[10] to send the annual Med: Register with my next Parcel of Books? I have not yet seen it, but shall of course turn to the article "Cowpox" with peculiar pleasure. Do you recollect my exhibiting some curious Pebbles, which I had collected during my stay in Town, to some Friends of yours in your apartment?[11] By some mishap, they were left behind me. They were good Specimens of Wood & Bone converted into Silex. I don't think there is a Corpuscle of the Globe we inhabit that has not breathed in the form of an animal or a vegetable. Adieu!

Believe me with best wishes   most truly Yours

Edwd. Jenner

Berkeley 9th Octobr. 1809

1. See Letters 38, 40, 46, and 51.

2. Dr. William Saunders, mentioned previously in Letters 38, 40, and 46. See also Letter 51 for the gift which Jenner sent to him.

3. The National Vaccine Establishment. See Letter 44.

4. The Right Honourable George Rose initiated the actions of Parliament which led to the founding of the National Vaccine Establishment. Sir Lucas Pepys, president of the College of Physicians of London, was also deeply involved. See Baron, *Life,* 2:117–24.

5. See Letter 31, n. 2.

6. The address of the Royal College of Physicians.

7. Sir Isaac Pennington. See Letter 38, n. 3.

8. M.T.C. [Thomas Charles Morgan], *An Expostulatory Letter to Dr. Moseley, on his review of the Report of the London College of Physicians on Vaccination* (London: printed for the author, and sold by J. Murray, 1808).

9. The wrapper of a letter or a postal packet.

10. W. Harwood was a bookseller at 21 Great Russell St. — *The Post-Office Annual Directory for 1813,* by Critchett and Woods, 14th ed. [London, 1813], p. 146.

11. It is of interest to note Jenner's use of the word "apartment" with evidently the same meaning as the current American usage. This was replaced in Britain by the Scottish term "flat" during the nineteenth century and is now obsolete in Britain.

50. To Dr. John Thomson, Halifax, 19 October 1809

Dear Sir[1]

I fear you must have felt hurt, or at least surpris'd at my silence after you had so long sent me your obliging Letter & the very excellent Pamphlet[2] which accompanied it. The fact is, I have not been at Cheltenham this season & they [di]d not reach me here till last night.

I know not when I have read anything on the Vaccine subject which has given me more satisfaction than your little Tract. It is exactly the kind of Thing I have long been wishing to see in circulation, as *all* who read it must understand it. The blows you have aim'd at those who still continue to inoculate the Smallpox, and the censure you pass on those deluded people who admit it into their families, I hope will [m]ake a due impression. Indiscrimin[a]te Inoculation may be consider'd as the grand source from which the Pestilence now draws its support. I have not been wanting in my endeavors to call the attention of the Legislature to the imm[en]se benefits the Empire would derive [fro]m their putting the present murderous System under due restrictions.[3] As "the safety of the Prince is in the People" why should a single life be thus wantonly wasted? No sooner were the doors of the Smallpox Hospital shut against Out-Patients, than others were open'd by many mercenary Apothecarys for this destructive business in various parts of the Metropolis. You justly observe if they could subdue the Smallpox in Ceylon why could no[t] the same thing be effected by the same m[e]ans here? This happy event has actually happen'd in districts more populous & extensive than Ceylon.

Your Tract I hope will find its way into every part of [ou]r dominions. Allow me to suggest the [pro]priety of your sending it to the Reviews — the most popular of the Magazines. I shall take care to distribute it largely here, where the people, from ten years absence of the Smallpox, begin to feel an apathy & neglect bringing the rising offspring for security. It strikes me that you have only seen the first & second parts of my early publications on the Cowpox. I should be happy to send you the third & some other papers, if you will tell me where they shall be left for you in London.

Believe me, dear Sir, with great respect, Your obliged & very faithful Servant

Edwd. Jenner

Berkeley — Glostre.
Octob: 19th 1809
Dr. Thomson   Halifax

1. John Thomson, graduated from Edinburgh in 1807, was a physician to the Halifax General Dispensary, corresponding member of the Literary and Philosophical Society of Manchester, and a former president of the Royal Medical Society of Edinburgh.

2. John Thomson, *Cheap tract on the cow-pox: A plain statement of facts, in favour of the cow-pox, intended for circulation through the middle and lower classes of society* (Halifax, 1809).

3. This was not achieved until 1840.

51.   To Dr. Thomas Charles Morgan, Dover, 31 December 1809

Berkeley
Decr. 31 1809

My dear Friend[1]

I need not tell you that I remain in the same lethargic kind of indolence, as when you heard from me last; my suffering your two friendly Letters to remain so long unanswered must convince you of it. I know your good heart would not allow you to put an uncharitable construction on my conduct. The Herrings came safe, & were facsimiles of those we feasted upon in your apartment in Town. Accept my best thanks for them. Game has been so scarce here this Season, that it has not been in my power to send you any.

I was sorry to find you had been destin'd again to visit Dover & be a resident there, of all places the most unlikely to make you happy. But the idea of the good you are doing among suffering humanity will act somewhat as a set off against unpleasant associations, & the up hill walk you are doom'd to take daily, will preserve your health. I wish I were compell'd to some exertion; left to my own voluntary choice, I go on moping. There is some excuse for me. My poor Boy still lives,[2] but without the most distant hope of recovery; and this idea ever haunts me. Stoical Philosophy is all nonsense — these People either possess'd no sensibility, or their real feelings were disguised by affectation. A man cannot change the nature of his mind at will, anymore than he can the colour of his Eyes. He must take it as it is presented to him & work it will, its own way.

Enclos'd is a Draft on my Banker for the discharge of Murray's Bill.[3] I not only pay it cheerfully, but with a thousand thanks to you for your kind exertions. Your excellent Letter certainly answer'd one good end — it convinc'd Moseley that he exposed himself by his absurdities. If he has stain'd a sheet of paper since, it has been done covertly. The opposition now seems to sleep — I hope my zealous Friend in New Street,[4] will not rouse them by any fresh *Scourge,* unless it should contain the excellent paper you gave him, which should certainly see the light. — Catherine[5] is now with me, grown tall & looking healthy. She & my family desire their best wishes to you. Mine will always attend you & your dear little Girl.

I have drawn the Bill a month after date, as from the nature of your engagements my Letter may not find you where it is directed to you. — Most truly Yours

Edw. Jenner

PS.   I am surpris'd at Dr. Saunders's[6] not receiving my Letters — One (a short one) was sent by Post & the other which occupied near four folio pages was put into a Basket with some Pheasants. As the Dr. never acknowledg'd rec'g the Game it is possible, neither one nor the other ever reach'd him. I hear little or nothing of the new Vaccine Establishment.[7] They will not benefit the Cause unless they adopt new plans & reputations —

1. See Letters 38, 40, 46, and 49. Morgan eventually became personal physician to John James Hamilton, the first Marquis of Abercorn, and moved to Ireland.

2. Edward Jenner, Jr., died from pulmonary tuberculosis two months later. See Letters 38, 46, 47, 49, 51, and 53.

3. In Letters 40 and 49 Jenner offered to pay the expenses for publishing Morgan's *Expostulatory Letter to Dr. Moseley,* which was printed and sold by J. Murray.

4. John Ring (see Letter 33), who had published *The Vaccine Scourge* anonymously. See Jenner's comments in Letter 38.

5. Jenner's daughter, at this time aged fifteen. On 7 August 1822 she married John Yeend Bedford, Esq., and died in childbirth on 1 August 1833. — Baron, *Life,* 2:289–90.

6. Dr. William Saunders, mentioned previously in Letters 38, 40, 46, and 49.

7. The National Vaccine Establishment. See Letter 44.

52.   To Thomas Paytherus, Esq., Great Russell St., Bedford Square, London, 16 January 1810

Berkeley Jan: 16 1810

Dear Paytherus[1]

At any other time than this I should make a long apology to you for suffering your first Letter to have remain'd [s]o long unanswer'd; but you know my situation, & believe me it is a very sad one, & unfits me for all kind of business.[2]

I don't exactly know the Spot you have fixt upon for your Family residence, but from some knowledge of the Country am assured it is a very pleasant one, & you have my hearty wishes that you & your's may enjoy it many years. Anything I can add to your Gardens you may command — The white Strawberrys, Catherine[3] shall bring on her return to Town — They are excellent, & produce Fruit three months in the year if the soil suit them. My red Strawberrys are only the common Alpine. As you are so near Cranford & L[or]d B. has let his Gardens you might furnish yourself with a variety of things there. I shall not let you alone till you have procured for me some of the Apple Trees that bear the *transparent Apples* such as you brought to your Table more than once last Summer twelve month. They seem to be a Breed from the Siberian Crab, but I suppose not Mr. Knight's. They would come safely by the Gloster Waggon with anything else, that is new & valuable from some of your choice Nurserys.

[12 lines crossed out]

I have not seen Maclean's Pamphlet,[4] & am therefore at a loss to know what shock the Triumvirate[5] you mention could have felt severe enough to loosen their hold from the emoluments of office, which they seem'd to grasp so tightly. Certain it is they are disgraced. Keat behaved most shamefully to me in the first House of Commons affair,[6] & Sr. Lucas' in the National Vac: Establishment[7] behaved in such a manner as to merit the same Epithet. Of the third, I have not much to say. Weir is a worthy man, & has talents; but I fear not a Constitution equal to the bustle of the office he has engaged in. It is with concern I see the cruel manner in which the family of Morse is treated by the present Ministry. The Brother who was at the War Office I find is dismiss'd. The ensuing Session will end their Career. It is to be lamented that it ever had a begining. The Gallic Emperor has shewn another specimen of his complaisance to me by listening to my petition & liberating two more British Captives from Verdun.[8] With all our best wishes to you & the Family, believe me truly Yours

Edw. Jenner

---

1. Thomas Paytherus, Esq., surgeon, of Ross-on-Wye near Berkeley was an old friend and colleague of Jenner's and a member of the Fleece Society (see Letter 17, n. 5). In 1800 he had published anonymously *A Comparative Statement of Facts and Observations Relative to the Cow-Pox; published by Doctors Jenner and Woodville* (London, 1800). In the second edition he admitted his authorship. (LeFanu 52, 53.)

2. Jenner's son, Edward, was dying from pulmonary tuberculosis.

3. Both Jenner's wife and daughter were named Catherine, but he always referred to his wife as "Mrs. Jenner."

4. Charles Maclean, *An Analytical View of the Medical Department of the British Army* (London, 1810). Charles Maclean, M.D. (fl. 1788–1824), had been in the service of the East India Company and had traveled extensively. He believed that epidemics were not contagious, that quarantine laws were futile, and he became a violent opponent of the government. In the summer and fall of 1809, a fruitless expedition against Napoleon's naval establishment at Antwerp had resulted in an enormous number of casualties from disease among troops on the Island of Walcheren. This led to a Parliamentary investigation. Maclean's pamphlet discussed the Walcheren expedition failure and criticized the medical department of the army.

5. The Medical Board of the Army, appointed politically, consisted of three members: Sir Lucas Pepys, the physician-general, Thomas Keate, Esq., the surgeon-general, and Francis Knight, Esq., inspector-general of hospitals. For the testimony of these three before the House of Commons, see *Gent. Mag.* 80 (1810): 262–63.

6. See Letter 39, n. 3.

7. Sir Lucas Pepys (1742–1830). See Letters 39 and 40.

8. Because of his internationally respected position, Jenner was frequently approached by his countrymen to use his influence in obtaining release of prisoners captured by Napoleon's armies (cf. also Letters 60, 65, and 66). In this instance Napoleon's favorite physician, Jean-Nicolas Corvisart (1755–1821), who was also actively promoting vaccination in France (cf. Letter A-9), served as Jenner's intermediary. See Baron, *Life,* 2:367, for another reference to this episode in a letter to James Moore.

53. To — — —, 26 February 1810

Berkeley 26th Feb: 1810

My dear Sir[1]

Before I notice the contents of your obliging Letter of the 20th instant, allow me to thank you for the very kind Epistle you address'd some time since to my Daughter & to unite her thanks with my own.

I shall be ever ready to come forward in the cause of Science. Mr. Cockerell[2] sha[ll] have any support in my power to afford him. The better way perhaps would be for you to send me a Certificate which should have my signature, & at the same time I would furnish him with a Letter, applauding his intentions, giving him my best wishes &c, &c.

You ask me for a popular Essay for the next Volume of the Memoirs of the Med. Society.[3] Oh my dear Sir, did you know the state of mind I am in at present, you would see how unfit I am for bringing out any literary production, or indeed for accomplishing scarcely anything. A few weeks since, I lost my eldest Son,[4] & the event has overwhelm'd me. You, from sad experience, know too well, what a Parent feels under such afflicting pressures. Whether, or when, I shall rise & be myself again, HE only knows who has cast me down. His will be done!

Adieu my dear Sir & believe me ever truly   Yours

Edwd. Jenner

March 8th

This Letter, short as it is, was begun, when dated on the other page —

1. The addressee is probably Dr. Alexander Marcet, originally from Geneva, who frequently served as a go-between for foreign visitors to London and for Englishmen traveling abroad. For other Marcet correspondence see Letter 7, n. 1.

2. Charles Robert Cockerell (1788–1863) became a leading British architect and art historian. In May 1810 he embarked on a tour of Greece, Asia Minor, and Sicily. — *Travels in Southern Europe and the Levant, 1810–1817: The journal of C. R. Cockerell, R.A.*, edited by his son, Samuel Pepys Cockerell (London, 1903); *DNB*.

3. Jenner is probably referring to the *Medico-Chirurgical Transactions* in which upon Marcet's solicitation he had published two papers in 1809. See Letter 37, 39, 41, 42, and 43.

4. Edward Jenner, Jr., died from pulmonary tuberculosis. See also Letters 38, 46, 47, 49, and 51.

54.   To Thomas Pruen, Esq., Woodbine Lodge, Cheltenham, 22 May 1810

Dear Pruen[1]

As opposite Bodies sometimes meet, I expected to have run against you at the Election, Friday. I had no conception that the Hero of M. Castle would have shewn the *White Feather* so hastily after declaring positively he would stand the Poll. What a Hurley-Burley for nothing, & what a shocking waste of Money! I think our young Senator, when Time has a little more matured his judgement, will not cut a bad figure in the House of Commons.

As Stibbs's Report respecting the Stables was favorable, I shall certainly accept of Mr. Newell's offer. The Money for payment is ready for him and he shall have a Draft as soon as I am put in possession of the Premises; or before if he wants it.[2]

Before the month of June is one third expired, I hope to be in London — stay a few days, & return with Catherine and Robert.[3] Then, if please God Mrs. Jenner's health & other circumstances will allow, I shall begin to think of going to Cheltenham, finish my deliberations in the *short* period of a month, & put my design in execution within a fortnight after.

Remember us kindly to Mrs. Pruen & believe me

Yours truly

Edw. Jenner

Berkeley
22 May 1810

PS.   This Letter was written some days since with the expectation of its being sent by Mr. Seager who promis'd to call here in his way from Bristol. I have seen your last Paper.[4] What has put Bob Hughes in such a Rage? The whole performance betrays a great want of political knowledge; but there is a little flippant sentence which has squeez'd itself in between two Brackets, for which I shall pick a Crow with him.

25 May

1. Thomas Pruen (ca. 1772–1834) was one of Jenner's close friends, who drifted from one profession to another during his life, beginning in the law and ending as a clergyman. The seventy-four letters written by Jenner to Pruen which are preserved at the Wellcome Historical Medical Library in London reveal that Jenner served as physician to the Pruen family and lent his friend money to support his newspaper-publishing activities. Pruen helped to promote vaccination, publishing *A comparative sketch of the effects of variolous and vaccine inoculation, being an enumeration of facts not generally known or considered but which will enable the public to form its own judgment on the probable importance of the Jennerian discovery* ([Cheltenham]: printed for Phillips, Crosby, Murray, Dwyer, and other Booksellers, 1807). Jenner relied upon Pruen to perform chores when he was absent from Cheltenham, such as having a piano shipped from Cheltenham to Berkeley and paying his insurance. An author of books on the history of chess and the liturgy of the Church of England, after Jenner's death Pruen expected to be his biographer. See Letter A-15, and also Letter 18, n. 2.

2. In the Jenner-Pruen correspondence there are frequent references to business matters of this nature, and Jenner sought Pruen's advice on how to install boilers in his new washhouse and how to remedy a smoking chimney. Thomas Newell (1763–1836), a surgeon, lived on the same terrace as Jenner. — Paul Saunders, *Edward Jenner: The Cheltenham Years, 1795–1823* (Hanover, N.H.: University Press of New England, 1982), p. 29.

3. Jenner's daughter and son.

4. *The Cheltenham Chronicle, and Glocestershire General Advertiser,* started by Pruen in May 1809. In a letter of 10 June 1810, Jenner advised him to get out from under the burden of the paper, which had run into financial difficulties. Pruen sold the paper in January 1811. In the same letter Jenner gives the following information about his own health: "My journey to Bath was solely for the purpose of a consultation of Physicians on my Case. It was agreed that my health had fallen into its present deranged state from reiterated agitations of my mind during a series of years in establishing Vaccination, and from the severe shock I lately experienced from another cause [his son's death]. My sentence is as follows. Cupping, blistering, purging, waterdrinking, a long Journey thro' untrodden regions, & a cessation of all mental con-

cerns. However, it is my intention to make one deviation, & before I make my tour, to go to Cheltenham as a probationary plan; & to be as quiet there as possible." — Edward Jenner to Thomas Pruen, 10 June 1810, Wellcome Historical Medical Library, London. There is no evidence that Jenner ever made the recommended tour for his health.

55. To Charles Murray, Esq., Bedford Row, London, 7 December 1810

My dear Sir[1]

It is very uncertain when I may visit London, but if my Friend Dr. Bateman[2] or any other Gentleman will have the kindness to be my Proxy, I shall with pleasure become responsible for my young Namesake's imbibing the rudiments of a Christian Education.[3]

I have seen the last Number of the Gent: Magazine, but Mr. Taylor's Letter does not appear.[4] I suppose it went too late; but the sooner Birch's[5] deceptions are put a stop to, the better. The same may be said of Maclean's & Moseley's.[6] This can't be done without some powerful Engine. But who is to construct it? One would think the statement of Facts, as they now stand before the Public from every quarter of the Globe would blow away such Stuff as these abominable People produce, like Chaff, but it is not so, or the Bills of Mortality would not exhibit weekly such horrid scenes of devastation from the Smallpox. The Legislature may perhaps be stimulated at the sight of this to take the Matter up. Indeed I think they ought as the Guardians not only of the property but the Lives of the Community. I think Mr. Wilberforce's philanthropy[7] would be rous'd into action, if he consider'd this matter; and who so proper to represent it to him as our Friend R. Phillips?[8]

I shall anxiously wait the result of your interview with Mr. J. Nicholls.[9] I cannot conceive the source of his hostility. Does he collect abuse as a more saleable commodity than its opposite? If so, what an atrocious Member of Society is John! In the Edinburgh Star of Friday Nov: 30th which I rec'd this day is an admirable report of Vaccination in opposition to Brown of Musselburgh.[10] You may probably get a sight of [i]t at some Coffee House. From a hint you once gave me it may be prudent to put my Friend Mr. Morris[11] in possession of my answer to Birch,[12] for I have not a doubt that Mr. Shaw Le Fevre[13] will introduce the subject in the House. It does not appear from your Letter that you have yet seen Maclean's Pamphlet.[14] I think myself Lawyer enough to say that it is a Libel meriting every severe Epithet lately pronounc'd against similar productions by L[or]d. Elenborough[15] & the Aty. Genl.

Make my best Comps. to Mrs. Murray & to Dr. Bateman for his good intentions. The enclosed Trifle, Mrs. Murray will be good enough to present to young Edward's Nurse.

Believe me,   Yours truly

Edw. Jenner

Cheltenham
7th Decemb: 1810

1. See Letters 34, 35, 58, and 62.

2. Thomas Bateman, M.D. (1778–1821), a pioneer in dermatology.

3. Jenner was accepting the office of godfather to Edward Jenner Murray, the sixth son of Charles Murray.

4. James Taylor's letter, addressed to "Mr. Urban" from Millman Place, 24 November 1810, was published in the December 1810 issue of *Gentleman's Magazine* (80, pt. 2:523–24). It was a reply to a letter signed "P.P." in the October issue (pp. 332–33).

5. John Birch had published a letter in the April 1810 issue of the *Gentleman's Magazine* (80, pt. 1:333–34) refuting an article in the April 1810 *Edinburgh Review*.

6. Charles Maclean (see Letter 52, n. 4) and Benjamin Moseley (Letter 18, n. 5) were both outspoken antivaccinists.

7. See Letter 44, n. 9.

8. See Letter 20.

9. John Nichols (1745–1826) was the editor of the *Gentleman's Magazine*. See also Letter 92.

10. Thomas Brown, surgeon of Musselburgh, had published *A Correspondence with the Board of the National Vaccine Establishment* (London, 1810).

11. Edward Morris, M.P. for Newport in Cornwall, had supported vaccination in 1807 by moving in the House of Commons that Jenner be awarded £20,000. See Baron, *Life*, 2:67–68.

12. Possibly the letter of 8 July 1808, published in *Gent. Mag.* 79 (April 1809): 315.

13. Charles Shaw Lefevre, M.P., president of the governors of St. Luke's Hospital, was an active antivaccinist in Parliament.

14. Charles Maclean, M.D., *On the State of Vaccination in 1810; in a letter to the right Hon. Richard Rider, His Majesty's Principal Secretary of State for the Home Department; with remarks on the Report of the National Vaccine Establishment. Printed by Order of the House of Commons, on the 1st of June, 1810. Forming a Guide for Parents in Deciding for the Safety of their Children* (London: printed for the author, 1810).

15. Edward Law (1750–1818), Lord Ellenborough, "that fountain of Rectitude and Virtue, the great Lord Chief Justice Ellenborough, of the King's Bench" (*Gent. Mag.* 80, pt. 2 [1810]: 508). The words are undoubtedly satirical, as he had many faults as a judge.

56. To William Lunell, Esq., Bristol, 5 January 1811

My dear Sir[1]

You need not be told how happy it would make me to render all the service in my power to Miss Wait, but unfortunately I shall be necessitated to remain at this Place, much beyond the period I had limited. Mrs. Jenner (who begs her kind remembrance to you) has been confin'd thro' one of her wintry indispositions for some weeks to her bed chamber, brought on by going to administer comfort to an afflicted poor Man, in a frosty day.

Now my good Sir, what shall we do? I am almost tempted to say, will not Miss Wait be benefited by a change of Scene, at least by that of changing the air of Bristol, a murky City, for the AEther of Cheltenham? Our Springs too might prove salubrious. In days of old you know, we could reckon but on one, now we boast of eleven. Our Chalybeate Spring rivals that of Tunbridge, and our Sulphurated Spa, the famous Water of the North. It is really a very extraordinary Fact, that all the Medicinal Waters of any celebrity in the Island are to be found concentrated in this little Spot, Bath excepted, & to this I attach no more value than that which flows from my Tea Kettle.

From the introductory part of your Letter, I see your Mind is as figurative as ever. I should like to crop a few of these poetic Flowers & put them into *Glasses;* of what kind you will not be long in guessing.

Pray make my respectful Comps. to the worthy Alderman & the Invalid, & thank them for the honor they intended me — and don't forget to present *our* kind remembrances to Mrs. Lunell & the Family.

Believe me truly   Yours

Edwd. Jenner

Cheltenham
5th Jany. 1811

1. See Letter 3.

57.   To Dr. Caleb Hillier Parry, Circus, Bath, 19 March 1811

My dear Friend [1]

Your Note address'd to me in Spring Gardens has found its way here. The Papers have since inform'd you of the suspension of the investigation for some time to come. During this interval every cruel engine which can be invented to torture the Berkeleys will be set to work. The Gloster Lawyers, whom we saw hovering about the Bar, are wandering in all directions to pick up any scrap of evidence that may tend to weaken the claim of L[or]d B. [2] I hope you did not suffer materially by your sudden call to Town. It will be my fate I fear to go again, as I have rec'd a kind of Demi-royal intimation to this effect. Another examination under circumstances so embarrassing as the last, would be the death of me. In an enquiry of such importance nothing could equal the carelessness of the Person who was appointed to shew me the Registers previously to my appearing before the House.

You may judge of the impression it has made, when I tell you that every night since, I have been summon'd to the Bar in my sleep and awoke trembling before the Wig of the Lord Chancellor. Such nerves as mine are not worth owning. Your Son Charles[3] sat an hour with me this morning. He is very well.

Believe me, my dear Friend   truly Yours

Edw. Jenner

Cheltenham
March 19 1811

1. See Letters 1, 14, and 17.
2. The fifth Earl of Berkeley, Frederick Augustus, had died the preceding August with Jenner, assisted occasionally by Parry, as medical attendant. The claims of Berkeley's eldest son, Col. William Berkeley, to the peerage were being examined by the Committee of Privileges of the House of Lords. Frederick Augustus had in 1796 married the daughter of a small tradesman by whom he had previously had several illegitimate children. In 1801 he attempted to legitimize these children by declaring that he had been secretly married in 1785. The evidence produced to prove this, a parish register entry, was clearly demonstrated by the committee of the House of Lords as having been a forgery. No judgment was given at this time, but in 1831 the eldest illegitimate son, Col. William Berkeley, who had retained tenure of the castle and lands, procured a peerage. — *Encyclopaedia Britannica*, 11th ed., s.v. "Berkeley."
3. See Letters 79, 80, 81, 90, and 91.

58.   To Charles Murray, Esq., Bedford Row, London, 22 September 1811

My dear Sir[1]

After the accounts you must lately have heard from this place respecting the health of poor Genl. Lyman[2] you will not be surpris'd at the doleful intelligence I now communicate. It was evident yesterday that he was in a dying state, & this afternoon at ten minutes past one, he expired without a groan or struggle. The Miss Lymans bear the loss with as much firmness as one can expect. I understand the family in Town will be appriz'd of the event by this Post.

The General's state of health continued nearly stationary from the time of his arrival here till the commencement of the late warm weather, soon after which he declined rapidly & another Tubercle burst about a week since, which discharged profusely.

Pray make my best Comps. to Mrs. Murray & Your Family & believe me very truly Your's

Edw. Jenner

Cheltenham
Sunday 3 o'Clock

1. See Letters 34, 35, 55, and 62. Undated by Jenner, this letter bears a postmark of 22 September 1811. This letter was published in Jacobs, "Edward Jenner," p. 751.

2. General William Lyman (1755–1811), a 1776 Yale graduate, had been a congressman and was appointed by Thomas Jefferson to serve as American consul and agent in London. He was buried in Gloucester Cathedral. After his death his daughters established a private school in Philadelphia. — Lyman Coleman, *Genealogy of the Lyman Family in Great Britain and America* (Albany, 1872), p. 453.

59. To Mrs. Cuming, [Cheltenham], 1 January 1812

Dear Madam

I am very sorry to find you are likely to have a return of your Cold. This is begining the New Year badly; but still I hope it may be the happiest that you and your family ever experienc'd. The Medicine which I directed for you at Albion House, was simply Paregoric Elixir & I have sent to Paytherus's to desire them to furnish you with some.

Miss T. Cuming, be assured, is not forgotten. She will have something to morrow.

I have the honor to be   with best wishes,   Dear Madam   Your obliged & obedient Servant

Edwd. Jenner

St. Georges Place, [Cheltenham]
New Year's day 1812

60. To Dr. Alexander J. G. Marcet, Russell Square, London, 26 March 1812

Berkeley March 26, 1812

My dear Doctor[1]

I cannot reply to your obliging Letters without an apology for what must appear to you an unwarrantable delay in the return of answers, & I must make the same to you as I am doom'd to make to many others. In fact the following is from necessity become a kind of Circular. Know then, my dear Friend, that I am extremely oppress'd by the variety & incessant operation of my Callings. Medical Men in general you know, however fully occupied, have the duties of their profession only to perform; but with regard to myself, I have as you well know the multifarious toils of Vaccination to attend to, the chief of which is a correspondence that knows no limits. This perplexes, indeed confuses me. For what can be more harrassing to the mind than a consciousness of having in one's possession heaps of unanswer'd Letters, while at the same time the generality of their authors are fill'd with amazement at my conduct from a misconception of its real cause. I cannot help further remarking that the duties of a Magistrate,[2] which during my residence at Berkeley I am compell'd to execute infringe not a little on that time, which I could wish to dedicate to other purposes.

I shall be extremely happy to put Mr. Stanhope's name on my List & to do all in my power for him should an opportunity present itself. But it would be wrong in me to flatter his Relatives with the expectation of my being able to do much, as the liberation of a british Captive has been very lately granted me, & I have another Petition before the French Government. Tho' I have some interest, yet you will see how slowly it operates, when I tell you that in the space of nine years I have been only able to bring away six Prisoners; and not one of these was a Military Man.[3] You will be shock'd to hear that our own Government refused at my solicitation to grant the release of a poor wounded young Officer, the Brother of Husson,[4] who has so often interested himself in my favor when making a similar request to the French Emperor. This was the more grating to my feelings as I was inform'd Mr. J. Kemble[5] did not ask in vain for the release of an officer who had the good luck to be the Brother of a French Comedian.

I am happy to hear the Medical Society[6] is in so flourishing a state, & tho' I have done so little yet I never lose sight of sending contributions. With respect to the Papers of which you so kindly sent me Copies, to confess the truth I have not yet look'd them over; but this you must attribute to the cause already assign'd for general delays.

I shall send for the Pamphlets, & anticipate much pleasure in the perusal, being confident you will find no difficulty in laying prostrate your Antagonist. But the worst of it is, he is so inflated with a light Gas, that he will get up again & hold his head as high as if he had never had a fall. "Hic niger est." How quickly our sagacious Friend Frank discover'd his *complexion.* I beg you to present my kind regards to Mrs. Marcet & my best wishes to the Stanhope Family & believe me, my dear Doctor most truly Yours

Edwd. Jenner

PS. If you will have the goodness to order Tilloch's Journalls[7] & with them the three last numbers of the *New* Medical Journal[8] from my Booksellers, Harwood, in great Russel Street, I should be obliged to you — He will send them by the Gloster Coach.

1. For other Marcet letters, see Letter 7, n. 1. Part of the first paragraph was published in Miller, "Letters," p. 13.
2. Justice of the peace. This was an unpaid position usually filled by the landed class of country gentlemen, whose duty it was to enforce the local laws and to maintain order. In Letter 77 Jenner discusses one of his cases with his son Robert.
3. A few details are in Baron, *Life*, 2:113–17. Jenner's role in the freeing of British prisoners of war was discussed in Letter 52, n. 8.
4. Henri-Marie Husson. See Letter 11. Further details about the attempt to free Captain Husson are in Letters 65 and 66. See also Baron, *Life*, 2:164–66.
5. John Philip Kemble (1757–1823), the well-known actor and manager of Covent Garden.
6. The Medical and Chirurgical Society of London.
7. The *Philosophical Magazine*, which had been established by Alexander Tilloch (1759–1825) in 1797 for the publication of new discoveries and inventions. An anonymous article in favor of vaccination was published in 1812 (39:152–54).
8. *New Medical and Physical Journal; or, Annals of Medicine, Natural History & Chemistry* had commenced in November 1810.

61. To Mr. Colnaghi, 23 Cockspur Street, London, 8 April 1812

Berkeley
April 8 1812

Sir[1]

I understand that the Gentleman who was kind enough to bring a Parcel for me from Milan is shortly about to return. My Packet for my Friend Dr. Sacco[2] is now ready or nearly so, and I should be happy to know when he returns & whether he would be good enough to take it with him to Milan? If so I should feel myself much obliged.

I am Sir   Your obliged & obedient Humble Servant

Edwd. Jenner

Please to direct to me at Berkeley Glostershire

1. *The Post-Office Annual Directory for 1813*, p. 71, lists Colnaghi & Co., "Picture & Caricature Merchants" at the Cockspur Street address. There were no government-sponsored international postal facilities at this time.
2. See Letter 38, n. 14.

62. To Charles Murray, Esq., Bedford Row, London, 25 September 1812

Cheltenham
Sunday

My dear Sir[1]

The information you communicate to me respecting Miss L.[2] fills me with astonishment. On her departure she gave a positive promise to come again to Cheltenham before she left England — I begg'd that the visit might be to us if we were there; if not that we might have the pleasure of receiving her & her Sisters at Berkeley. The invitation was accepted & I cannot help thinking that she intended coming as there are at this moment a considerable number of Letters directed for her at my House, & are now remaining at Berkeley, forwarded from the Post office here. I went from hence with my family about three weeks since, but am come back again on medical business. On Wednesday or Thursday I purpose returning. Before I close this I shall make an enquiry at the late General's Lodging whether everything is settled, & whether any debt remains elsewhere.

The Annual Report of the R. V. Establishment[3] is likely to be a good one I hear, & that the new President conducts the business of the Institution with ardor. I am happy to hear this. Something was certainly wanted to make up for the languid proceedings of his Predecessor. When you write again will you have the kindness to name to me the Gentlemen who compose the present Board? I have lately sent many Documents — Mr. Moore[4] ask'd for De Carro's Report[5] — I have not had one since that inserted in your Pamphlet.[6] Pearson's[7] last Report should be burnt by the common Hangman for its insinuation respecting Eruptions. — It will murder thousands. Pray speak to Mr. Moore & refer him to De Carro, if he intends inserting an extract; but it should be observed that this is rather stale & has been a good deal hacknied.

Tuesday

I have now finish'd my enquiry here respecting Miss L. & as far as I can learn nothing remains unsettled. The person where the Family lodged informs me that they pass'd thro' Cheltenham in their way to Liverpool.

Believe me, my dear Sir,   Very sincerely Your's

Edw. Jenner

If you should chance to see my Friend Phillips[8] in the Poultry[9] pray thank him for his kind attention to me in sending his Publications &c &c &c. I *mean* to write to him.

[The following names appear, evidently in Jenner's handwriting, on the outside fold:] Dr. Pemberton   D. Dundas

           Frumpton   T. Forster

           Ash   E. Home

           Cooke

1. See Letters 34, 35, 55, and 58. The date is given by the postmark.

2. Miss Lyman. See Letter 58, n. 2.

3. The National Vaccine Establishment. See Letter 39, n. 3, and also Letters 40–42, 44, 45, and 49 for Jenner's early difficulties with it. The new president was Sir Francis Milman. Jenner supplied many of the documents for the report. — Baron, *Life,* 2:182 ff.

4. James Moore, Esq., a surgeon, was the director of the National Vaccine Establishment. See Letter 73, n. 2.

5. Jean de Carro of Vienna. See Letter 5. De Carro sent reports to Jenner of the progress of vaccination in India and other parts of the world.

6. Charles Murray, *An answer to Mr. Highmore's objections to the Bill before Parliament . . . with an appendix containing some interesting communications from foreign medical practitioners on the progress and efficacy of vaccine inoculation* (London, 1808).

7. George Pearson, M.D. (1751–1828), Jenner's old enemy. See Letter 17, n. 2.

8. Richard Phillips (1767–1840), author, bookseller, and publisher. See Letter 20.

9. A London street with numerous bookshops.

63. To Dr. Alexander J. G. Marcet, Russell Square, London, 26 September 1812

My dear Doctor[1]

Permit me to introduce to you a young Friend of mine, Mr. Dunning from Plymouth, who is come to Town to attend your Hospital.[2] I am under very great obligations to his Father[3] who early enlisted into the Vaccine Corps & has long since become, like yourself, a General in the antivariolous army! Young Dunning has no acquaintances or Friends in Town, & therefore any little attention you might be good enough to shew him would be gratefully recollected, not only by him & the family, but by myself also.

I have not been at Cheltenham this Season, but have spent the summer at my Cottage at Berkeley, not in idleness, believe me. We talk of Chronic inflammation of the Liver. This is vague kind of language — How it commences, what system of Hepatic Vessells it first attacks, how it makes its progress & leads on to Scirrhus, has not, as far as I know, been yet explain'd. I think I have made something out. But perhaps this has been already done by others & my labors are useless. This you must tell me. If my observations should be new & correct, a Paper on the Subject may be acceptable to our Society for their next Volume.[4] I will just mention that there are two causes of scirrhosity each having a distinct source; the one arising from Hydatids, the other from inflammation of the internal Coats of the biliary Ducts. My observations have been drawn from the dissection of diseas'd Quadrupeds; but the general appearance of the Liver & its effects in exciting other diseases; particularly Hydrothorax, will not I believe be found to differ from the human.

I do not despair of shaking you by the hand in Russel Square before Winter commences. Pray make my kindest regards to Mrs. Marcett & believe me, my dear Doctor, with great respect, very truly Your's

Edwd. Jenner

Berkeley
Sept: 26th 1812

1. For other letters to Marcet, see Letter 7, n. 1.
2. Marcet had been appointed physician to Guy's Hospital in 1804.
3. Richard Dunning, a Plymouth surgeon, was one of Jenner's earliest supporters. In his pamphlet *Some observations on vaccination* (London, 1800) he had introduced the words *vaccination* and *vaccinate*. — LeFanu, p. 50. As surgeon and secretary to the Dock Jennerian Institution in 1804 he had published *Minutes of some experiments to ascertain the permanent security of vaccination against exposure to the small-pox. To which are prefixed some remarks on Mr. Goldson's pamphlet. With an appendix containing testimonials and other communications* (Dock [Plymouth], 1804) and in 1805 *Further observations on the practice of vaccination* (Dock, 1805). In 1802 Dunning, writing in behalf of the Medical Society of Plymouth, persuaded Jenner to sit for a portrait by James Northcote which is now in the possession of the Plymouth Medical Society. — LeFanu, p. 158. Fifteen letters from Jenner to Dunning are printed in Baron's *Life,* 2:330–59.
4. The Medical and Chirurgical Society of London. There is no evidence that Jenner ever wrote this article.

64. To Mr. Robert Jenner, c/o Rev. J. Joyce, Henley, Oxon, 2 December 1813

My dear Robert[1]

On Monday last I sent you a Letter enclosing two Notes for a Guinea each. It was more than once stipulated between us that every Letter containing Bills should be answer'd by return of Post. What makes me the more fearful that my Monday's Letter has miscarried is Mr. Ferryman's[2] calling here this morng. who I find had an interview with you yesterday, & his not saying anything about it tho' we rec'd the Parcel you sent by him. We should have been extremely happy to have heard by him that you were looking well, but we were griev'd to hear that you look'd pale & thin. When you left us, you were stout & in good health. Pray tell me, are you entirely free from Cough, or Complaints about your Chest of any sort of kind? Such as a sense of tightness or difficult breathing on using any great exertion? Have you at any time a pain in your side under the Ribs? Are your bowels got back to the old state of costiveness? Don't fail to tell me, if you are unwell the precise feelings you experience.

I trust you diligently attend to all I have said again & again about cold. The Post is going out & I can only add with what anxiety & affection I remain truly Yours

E.J.

Thursday near 6 o'clock P.M.
[*Post office stamp:* Dec. 2, 1813 Cheltenham]

1. Robert Fitzharding Jenner (1797–?), the second son of Edward Jenner, whose unsuccessful vaccination at the age of eleven months is recorded in Jenner's *Inquiry into the Causes and Effects of the Variolae Vaccine* (London, 1798), pp. 40–41. At this time he was away at school, preparing to matriculate at Oxford. He became a career army officer and never married. Beginning with sentence four, this letter has been published in Jacobs, "Edward Jenner," p. 749. See also Letters 71, 75, 77, 78, and 97.

2. The Reverend Robert Ferryman, an old friend and vaccination ally, who had architectural interests and built the summer house, the "Temple of Vaccinia," in Jenner's garden at Berkeley. For an effusive description of this "rustic apartment" where Jenner vaccinated his poor neighbors, see Baron, *Life*, 2:297–98, and Thomas Dudley Fosbroke, *Berkeley Manuscripts* (London, 1821), pp. 227–28. Jenner wrote as follows of Ferryman in a letter to Thomas Pruen: "I have just got a Letter from Ferryman. He says if he could get a Curacy he would relinquish his Post at Hallifax. Do you happen to know of a vacancy. He dates his Letter from the Cove of Cork. What a strange jumble of intellect does this unfortunate man possess. How much he has mistaken himself, & put that in front which should have been in the background. He is preeminent (in my opinion) as a Landscape Gardener & by pursuing this for the benefit of others, he might have enrich'd himself — but he must become an Architect & be hanged to him, ruin himself & those who were heedless enough to employ him." — Letter of 19 December 1817, Wellcome Historical Medical Library, London.

65. To Richard Dobson, [Hospital Ship Trusty], Chatham, [December, 1813]

To Dr. Dobson[1]
Chatham
"There is among the French Prisoners of War under your inspection on board one of the ships at Chatham, an Officer of the name of Husson.[2] From a variety of circumstances I feel myself much interested about this young Man. He is the Brother of my particular Friend Doctr. Husson a distinguished Physician at Paris.

I have had the happiness of liberating many of the british Captives & restoring them to their Families and Friends; and in furthering the object of my Petitions to the French Govt., I had always the ready assistance of Dr. Husson. It was therefore natural for him when the chance of War threw his Brother on our Shores, to look to my exertions for his liberation. I felt an exultation I freely own at the application, not conceiving, after the benefits our Fleets & Armies had derived from my labors, that my solicitation would have been rejected; especially too as it was the first I had made in behalf of a French Prisoner.

Without troubling you with detail, I shall only briefly remark that at the onset of this business, I had every prospect of being successful and I firmly believe that my communicating this to Capt. Husson laid the foundation for his present sufferings. He was of course elated at it; but I was soon compell'd to let him know that my efforts were unavailing. He fell into despondency, and under its pressure broke his Parole.

My request to you, Sir, then is this — to exercise your humanity towards him in any way that circumstances will admit — by cheering him with your conversation & assuring him that bad as his prospects are, he is not to despond for I shall still persevere in my efforts to obtain his liberation.

It has often been reported to me that he was in very ill health, that he was maim'd in different actions on the continent & that he still suffer'd from his wounds. If this be really the case & he would no longer be of use to the armies of his Country, might he not on this plea be restored to his Friends from your Report? I ask this question with deference. I should observe that our Government will allow me to exchange him for an Officer of equal rank from France, provided the French Government will accede to the arrangement, but I fear there are many obstacles in the way of it.

I beg pardon for this intrusion & have the honor to be &c &c

Edwd. Jenner

1. Richard Dobson (ca. 1773–1847) was a prominent naval surgeon who in 1814 became surgeon at the Royal Marine Infirmary at Chatham and in 1824 surgeon to Greenwich Hospital. He obtained an M.D. degree from St. Andrews in 1824 and was knighted in 1831. Dobson replied to this letter on 23 January 1814, according to Jenner's letter of 16 February 1814 to Dobson, published in W. W. Francis and Lloyd G. Stevenson, "Three Unpublished Letters of Edward Jenner," *Journal of the History of Medicine and Allied Sciences* 10 (1955): 365–66.

Although in Jenner's handwriting, this document appears to be a copy of Jenner's original letter to Dobson, since it contains no salutation and the closing is incomplete. In addition, quotation marks are found at the beginning of the first sentence.

2. Captain Husson, the brother of Henri-Marie Husson, the French promoter of vaccination (see Letters 11, 66, and A-9), had been a prisoner of war since July 1808. For details see Baron, *Life,* 2:164–66.

66.   To Dr. Henri-Marie Husson, Paris, 13 December 1813

My dear Sir[1]

I want to write to you on a great variety of subjects among which Vaccination will form a principal feature. I want to express to you the great obligations which you & many of my Confreres in France have plac'd me under; but all must be postpon'd for the present.

The Packet which brings you this, will convey a Petition to the Emperor for the liberation of Capt. Milman;[2] and the chief of my present concise Letter is to assure you, that from the *certain knowledge* which I have of the intentions of our Government, I am enabled to pledge *myself fully,* that as soon as Cpt. Milman arrives in England, Captain Husson will be allow'd to return to France.[3]

Believe me, dear Sir,   with every sentiment of regard   Most sincerely Yours

Edwd. Jenner

Berkeley   Gloucestershire   Decr. 13 1813
Dr. Husson   Paris

1. See Letters 11 and A-9. Jenner discussed the difficulties he was having in obtaining the release of Husson's brother in Letters 60 and 65.
2. Captain Milman was a son of Sir Francis Milman (1746–1821), who had been president of the Royal College of Physicians and was physician in ordinary to the king.   — W. W. Francis and Lloyd G. Stevenson, "Three Unpublished Letters of Edward Jenner," *Journal of the History of Medicine and Allied Sciences* 10 (1955): 363; *DNB,* 13:448.
3. Jenner's letter of 16 February 1814, published by Francis and Stevenson, shows that Milman was released by Napoleon at this time; presumably Husson was freed immediately thereafter.

67.   To Dr. Richard Worthington, Southend near Upton, 20 December 1813

My dear Doctor[1]

I am suddenly summon'd to the Inkstand by a report that Mrs. Hyde intends setting off to-morrow morning for Southend. Little did I think, *whatever you did,* that after suffering your servant to depart without an answer to your Letter, that I should have so long remain'd mute. It griev'd me to hear that your Journey into the North turn'd out a melancholy one. But we must murmur as little as our nature will allow us at these decrees knowing from whose *fiat* they come. My poor dear Robert[2] came home from School about ten days since with a bad Cough & looking so peculiarly ill, so like his lost Brother, that I was almost struck dead at his appearance. Thank God! he is already much better & his Cough nearly gone. Our sheet Anchor in threatening Cases I believe is the constant breathing of air duly regulated as to temperature. One very cheering circumstance is, his not having a quick pulse.

I hope you have all escaped the Catarrh of the day, or gone thro' it in a moderate way. It has been very general here & in many instances very severe. Your motion respecting the Preface to the Worcester Eulogy I beg leave to second; it will come in very well. I went to Oxford last week to receive my Honors & met with a warm reception there.[3] There is one good shews itself in their coming so late. It proves that the Judgement of the University was fully matured as to the merits of Vaccination. There is another thing for consideration. The Degree of Doctor in Medicine by *Diploma* is a Boon that has not been bestow'd on any man for near a Century before.

You will think me miserably parsimonious in the manner your generosity to Mr. Rowlands is repaid when you open the enclos'd packet; but the truth is, you nearly share with me my precious stock. I kept the Cow till she died from age. I had a Calf & that was cut off prematurely. The Hair grew on the Tail of the Cow that infected the Dairy Girl, Sarah Nelmes from whose hand the Matter was taken that spread Vaccination thro' the World. (see my first Treatise)[4] The Cow was *Gloster* with a dash of the northern, & a famous milker.[5] I am quite in love with the Flanders Pippin[6] & must have (not for love but money) half a dozen more grafted Stocks sent to Berkeley, besides a good bundle of Grafts, in due season.

I have tried bark[7] for a Case of head ache similar to your good Lady's accompanied with Bronchocele, but my recollection does not furnish me with one. This is no reason why Mr. Rowlands should be correct & I trust that the Headache & the Tumor may go off together.

How did your green Ribbons, the other day, like the Thermometer at 16°? Did they not in compliment to the times assume the tint of orange or was this reserv'd for the *Carpet-weaving* Farmer?[8] Young Ladies are generally so fond of young Music, that I know not how Miss Worthington will relish what I have sent her — as it is as old as Wm. Shakespear. With the best regards of myself & Family, believe me, my dear Doctor

Most truly Your's

Edw: Jenner

[*In another hand:*] Memorand. Apple Cuttings for Dr. Jenner

1. The Reverend Dr. Richard Worthington (M.D. Edinburgh 1778), born in Shropshire, was an intimate friend who had advised Jenner to publish his *Inquiry* privately after it was rejected by the Royal Society. See LeFanu, p. 24. Part of this letter was published in Jacobs, "Edward Jenner," p. 750, and in Miller, "Letters," pp. 16–17. See also Letter 83. Other letters to Worthington are in Baron, *Life,* 2:405–10, 412–14, 417–18. E. G. Salisbury, *Border Counties Worthies,* 1st ser. (London, 1880), p. 302, describes Worthington as "a man of mark, a scholar, a good writer, and above all a true patriot, who desired to render moral and spiritual service to his countrymen, at a time when revolutionary opinions were undermining the foundations of society."

2. His son Robert Fitzharding Jenner. See Letters 64, 71, 75, 77, 78, and 97.

3. This is described in detail by John Baron, who accompanied him from Cheltenham to Oxford on 14 December 1813. See Baron, *Life,* 2:189–90.

4. *An Inquiry into the Causes and Effects of the Variolae Vaccinae, a Disease Discovered in Some of the Western Counties of England, Particularly Gloucestershire, and Known by the Name of the Cow Pox* (London, 1798).

5. The Henry Barton Jacobs Collection of the Welch Medical Library possesses some of the hair from this cow's tail.

6. A variety of apple.

7. Peruvian bark, or Cinchona.

8. Worthington carried on extensive farming activities which are referred to in Jenner's other letters to him.

68.   To Dr. Hamel, Count Orloffs, Upper Seymour Street, London, 13 May 1814

My dear Sir[1]

I should be very happy to introduce you to Dr. Baillie[2] & Mr. Cline.[3] I dined with Dr. Baillie yesterday, & took the opportunity of mentioning the subject & he beg'd me to give you an invitation to join a Party at his House on Thursday evening next. As it is my intention to be there, I can then introduce you.

I have at last procured a House, No. 7 Great Marylebone Street, where I should be happy to see you. I commonly breakfast soon after nine o'clock & shall be always glad to see you as one of my Party.

Yours my dear Sir   very truly

Edw. Jenner

Friday morning
13 May 1814

1. Count Orloff was Russian ambassador to the British court, and Dr. Hamel was his medical attendant. Dr. Hamel is also mentioned in Thomas Dudley Fosbroke, "Biographical Anecdotes of Edward Jenner," in *Berkeley Manuscripts* (London, 1821), p. 240. See also Letter 69.

2. Matthew Baille (1761–1823), anatomist, nephew of John Hunter, and physician extraordinary to George III.

3. Henry Cline (1750–1827), prominent surgeon, student of John Hunter, became president of the Royal College of Surgeons. — Sir William MacCormac, *An Address of Welcome delivered on the Occasion of the Centenary Festival of the Royal College of Surgeons of England* (London: Ballantyne, Hanson & Co., 1900), pp. 58–61.

69. To Dr. Hamel, Count Orloffs, Upper Seymour Street, London, [1814]

Thursday Evening

My dear Sir[1]

Are you alive, or were you drown'd in the Storm after I left you Wednesday morning? If you are in the land of living pray come & take your Breakfast with me tomorrow morning.

Be good enough to tell Dr. Meyer that I executed his commission, but have received no answer.

Yours truly

Edw: Jenner

1. See preceding Letter 68. Although this letter bears no date, it was unquestionably written in 1814, the last time Jenner resided in London from the end of April until midsummer. For details see Fisk, *Dr. Jenner,* pp. 255–57. Baron, *Life,* 2:205 ff, implies that Jenner took up residence in London in order to be present during the June visit of the victorious anti-Napoleonic leaders following the defeat of the First Empire and the signing of the Treaty of Paris on 30 May 1814.

70. To Dr. Alexander J. G. Marcet, Russell Square, London, [16 May 1814]

My dear Friend[1]

Your obliging Note has pursued & overtaken me in the Street. Of all things I should like to be of your party today, but alas, previous engagements are obstacles not to be removed. I am sorry it so happens. We shall meet I hope soon somewhere.

Most truly Your's

Edwd. Jenner

Charing Cross
Monday Noon.

1. See Letter 7, n. 1. The date was added in another hand.

71. To Mr. Robert Jenner, Mr. Joyces, Henley, Oxon, 18 June 1814

Dear Robert[1]

You would not have had another Letter so soon had it not been for your telling me that your Cough still continues. In my opinion you cannot have recourse to the remedy too soon; however at all events call on Dr. Routh.[2] The sort of Cough you had when here, is sometimes more troublesome to cure, & is apt to continue longer when it attacks at once with greater severity.

Your gratification with regard to our great foreign Guests[3] must be now complete. I went to see the renown'd Platoff[4] yesterday & found him in bed, or rather lounging there wrapp'd in a Pelise. He is a very interesting Figure & tho' he rose from low rank to the dignity of *Hetman*,[5] is full of politeness. His Countenance has a good deal of the Calmuck[6] in it. His Snuff was very excellent.

I have been to the Oldenburgh Hotel no less than three times by the command of the Emperor & Grand Duchess, & was detain'd many hours each time for no purpose. Such Confusion, & such a Medley of Cossacs, Moldavians, Greeks & all sorts of english I never saw before.[7]

You shall hear again   Your affectionate Father

E. Jenner

The Postman waits
Saturday

1. See Letters 64, 75, 77, 78, and 97. The second and third paragraphs were published in Miller, "Letters," p. 16.

2. Unidentified.

3. These included the Russian czar Alexander I, his sister the grand duchess of Oldenburg, King Frederick William III of Prussia, and Field Marshal Gebhard Leberecht von Blücher. In a letter to his friend Thomas Pruen dated 14 May 1814, Jenner described his activities further: "My visit to the Metropolis at this time, was in obedience to many calls of consequence. The Court had a demand upon me, & there I have been, made up of shreds and patches like a Morris Dancer — My Friend Andrews furnish'd me with his Carriage on this grand occasion. Another object was to pay my devoirs to some of the great Russians already come, & those who are coming. I have been closeted for more than an hour with one who was worth going to Kamschatka to see, her Imperial Highness the grand Duchess of Oldenburgh. She is by far the first woman of a Royal Race I have ever met with." —Jenner-Pruen Correspondence, Wellcome Historical Medical Library, London.

4. Matvei Ivanovich Platov (1751–1818), general of the cavalry of the Don Cossack Host, became a hero for his actions against Napoleon. He received an Oxford honorary doctorate during this visit. — *Great Soviet Encyclopedia*, trans. of 3rd ed. (New York: Macmillan, 1979).

5. A cossack headman.

6. Kalmucks were members of Buddhist Mongol tribes who had formerly lived on the lower Volga.

7. These meetings are described in detail in Thomas Dudley Fosbroke, "Biographical Anecdotes of Dr. Jenner," in *Berkeley Manuscripts* (London, 1821), pp. 236–40.

72. To Dr. Alexander J. G. Marcet, Russell Square, London, [23 June 1814]

My dear Doctor[1]

Do you recollect the interchange of a promise at Sir W. Farquhars,[2] to go some day & see our Friend Dr. Saunders?[3] Either Sunday or Monday would suit me; & if either of these days would be agreeable to you, you have only to tell me at what hour I should call for you.

Perhaps Mrs. Marcet would not dislike a little country oxygen. We should then be just the right number for *Chemical conversations.*[4]

Truly Your's

Edwd. Jenner

7 Great Marylebone St.
Wednesday Night

1. See Letter 7, n. 1. The date is in another hand.
2. Sir Walter Farquhar (1738–1819), M.D. Aberdeen in 1796, was physician in ordinary to the Prince of Wales.
3. William Saunders, M.D. (See Letter 38, n. 10). He was the first president of the Medical and Chirurgical Society and is mentioned in Letters 38, 40, 46, 49, and 51. He lived at Enfield from 1814 until his death in 1817.
4. Jane Marcet had published *Conversations on Chemistry, intended more especially for the Female Sex* in 1806.

73. To Dr. Alexander J. G. Marcet, Russell Square, London, 24 June 1814

My dear Friend[1]

Pray come & breakfast with me tomorrow morning. A Friend or two will meet you.

Mr. J. Moore[2] wishes for a list of the Medico Chirurgical Society[3] — Will you have the kindness to put one in your Pocket?

Ever Yours

E. Jenner

7 Gt. Marylebone St.
Friday afternoon

1. See Letter 7, n. 1. The date is indicated in the postmark.

2. James Moore, Esq., was surgeon to the 2nd Regiment of Life Guards and director of the National Vaccine Establishment. A faithful friend, he kept Jenner informed of current activities related to vaccination and wrote two books, *The History of the Smallpox* (London, 1815), dedicated to Jenner, and *The History and Practice of Vaccination* (London, 1817). A number of letters from Jenner to Moore are published in Baron, *Life,* 2:126–28, 361–404.

3. See Letter 23, n. 11.

74. To Dr. Alexander J. G. Marcet, Russell Square, London, [3 July 1814]

My dear Doctor[1]

That you may not be disappointed, I send this to say I have engaged some Friends to breakfast with me tomorrow morning. I shall leave Town Monday[2] & not without regret at being deprived of the pleasure of witnessing your curious Experiment.

In the course of tomorrow, if I can by any means steal an hour & get into a Fiacre, I certainly will pay a visit to Mrs. Mallit.

I seiz'd upon the little Tube as soon as it arriv'd & expos'd it to the heat of a Candle, but I could not bring your violet into Blossom. I was afraid to give it a strong heat & perhaps the failure was owing to this. Once more then, & for the last time, let me tax your pen & Ink two minutes to tell me how I must manage this curious Hot house plant.

Farewell my dear Doctor — Most sincerely Your's

Edwd. Jenner

Saturday Night
7 Great Marylebone Street

1. See Letter 7, n. 1. The date is in another hand.
2. This was Jenner's last sojourn in London.

75. To R. F. Jenner, Esq., Exeter College, Oxford, 23 April 1815

Dear Robert[1]

Your first Letter giving me an account of your arrival in Oxford in *good time,* afforded me much pleasure; but that of yesterday was still more pleasant as it delights me to find that you are enlisted in the scientific ranks of Professor Buckland.[2] Be assured Robert, that whatever your mind imbibes of this description will be of lasting benefit & will, as you advance in life, afford you more real & substantial gratification than thousands of those baubles which you have frequently [been] seeking for, and which, if they have been brought within your grasp, what are they? Bubbles, no sooner form'd than burst & gone. I hope you will take some Notes on anything particularly interesting that Mr. Buckland developes, especially with regard to *our* Rocks.

I have not seen or heard anything of Mr. Ferryman[3] in this part of the World, & of course am still without the Lettuce Seed. Having obtain'd a promise of Garden seeds from the South of Spain & from Genoa, I am in hopes they may arrive time enough for sowing; but the Season is advancing. The fruit Trees in most Gardens blossom vigorously — The present long continued wet weather I fear will be injurious. Rain is now falling, & it has continued to rain incessantly near forty hours. I suppose Catherine[4] in her Letter told you that Mr. H. Hicks's[5] present of a Horse (tho' a *Monoc*)[6] is likely to be very useful to her.

We did not forget your Birthday; but it was not kept with any particular festivity as I find it was your wish this might be reserv'd till your return.

Poor Harriet[7] still lingers on. A swelling has at length appear'd in her side which affords us a shadow of hope, & but a shadow.

I have done nothing yet with respect to Cheltenham — the unfortunate business at Kingscote & a vast influx of Letters foreign & domestic deranged my plans in such a way that I know not what to do — and I have no assistance from any quarter whatever, except what I derive in the practical part of Vaccination from Friends' Hands.

Dear Robert   Your affectionate Father

Edw. Jenner

I shall mention to H. Shrapnell[8] what you desire me — Your Letters come a day sooner via Dursley.

Berkeley 23d April 1815

1. See Letters 64, 71, 77, 78, and 97.
2. Prof. William Buckland (1784–1856), noted Oxford geologist, was professor of mineralogy.
3. See Letter 64, n. 2.
4. Jenner's daughter.
5. See Letter 8, n. 3.
6. Probably monoculate, or one-eyed.
7. Probably Harriet Kingscote, the sister of Sir Henry Peyton, who had married Thomas Kingscote, the brother of Jenner's wife, in 1794. She was still living at Kingscote in 1821. — Thomas Dudley Fosbroke, *Berkeley Manuscripts* (London, 1821), pedigree of Kingscote facing p. 218.

8. Henry Shrapnell, a surgeon, became a younger partner of Jenner and took care of his natural history collections. — Fisk, *Dr. Jenner,* pp. 174, 261.

76. To Dr. Thomas Harrison Burder, 27 Southampton Row, Russell Square, London, 5 February 1816

My dear Sir[1]

Accept my best thanks for your kind attention. Had I known that so heavy a task had been impos'd on you, & that you were suffering under indisposition my request would probably have been withheld. As you have been good enough to accomplish it, I will trouble you to forward your Papers made up into a Packet by the Gloucester Mail Coach directed for me at Berkeley Glostershire.

I quitted Cheltenham soon after the doleful event had taken place[2] & am now residing at my house here, as a public place by no means harmonizes with the present state of my feelings. These privations, my dear Sir, cut deep, and in a mind possess'd of sensibility, produce sensations of the most painful kind. You point to a source of the highest consolations, & I feel grateful to every friend who thus exhibits a feeling Heart. There is a secret Charm in sympathy — How soothing is it to the wounded Spirit.

You speak of your engagements — I hope they are of a nature to afford you pleasure & that professional calls are already occupying part of your time, as a reward for your attentions & laborious exercises during your long residence in Scotland.[3] I could wish you for a moment to turn to your Notes on the Lymphatics & just tell me whether anything new is said of their structure — If I recollect right, a lymphatic has two Coats, the external less delicate than the internal.

Believe me with best wishes   dear Sir   very truly Yours

Edw. Jenner

Berkeley
Feb: 5th 1816

Pray remember me to my old Friend Mr. Blair[4] when you see him.

[*Note in pencil in another hand:*] Dr. Jenner is full of humanity. He had lately lost Mrs. Jenner, who was considered to be a pious woman, & had, I believe, ascribed her religious impressions to the Village Sermons.

1. Thomas Harrison Burder (d. 1843) obtained his M.D. degree at Edinburgh in 1815. The last paragraph of this letter was published in Jacobs, "Edward Jenner," p. 752. The letter contains a black mourning seal.

2. Jenner's wife Catherine (Kingscote) had died on 13 September 1815. — Baron, *Life,* 2:220. After returning to Berkeley, Jenner never left again, except for a day or so.

3. Burder had been studying medicine at the University of Edinburgh.

4. William Blair. See Letters 44 and 45.

77. To Robert Fitzharding Jenner, Esq., Exeter College, Oxford, 17 February 1816

Berkeley Sat: night
Feby. 17 1816

My dear Robert[1]

In complyance with your request I have sent enclos'd a Draft on Ladbroke[2] for 20 drawn in the way you desire.

I am quite shock'd to think you have such a wretched apartment. Cold indeed it must have been for water almost upon the fire to have frozen in it. A pleasant change has now taken place in the weather & I trust the frosty part of the winter has nearly ceas'd; but among us medical men, the month of March is considered as the most trying to a second rate Constitution, such as yours, in the whole year, and while Time is maturing your mind, you will feel more & more forcibly, the reiterated admonitions you have received from me on this important subject & not treat it lightly, at least I trust you will. By attention to this, & the management of your Stomach you will give firmness & durability to a frame which from heedlessness to these important points, must soon sink & lie prostrate in the dust.[3]

You tell me you have not been quite so well since the cold weather has set in. This vague mode of making the communication fills me with anxiety & suspence & I must entreat you, if ever you should have occasion to speak on so unpleasant a subject again, that you will be explicit. I shall of course hear from you immediately, & be impatient to know the nature of your complaint. Your Grocery scheme may do well enough, but that respecting wine cannot be judicious. It would be perfectly so were you settled & a Housekeeper; but a stock of Wine the property of an undergraduate could not from the nature of Things, remain a stock long. Depend upon it, in a place like Oxford, there are wines in the Merchants' Cellars always to be had in a state of maturity if you seek for them thro' proper Channels. Dr. Kidd,[4] Sir Christopher,[5] Dr. Wall,[6] or any of my Friends would direct you how to procure them. You know at Cheltenham, I can obtain this from several of the Wine Merchants just as good from their Vaults as if it had lain in my own. Never, then, would I lay in more than a Hamper at a time. Be assured I do not mean that you should purchase an inferior sort, the common College trash; tho' the only difference is that one destroys the Constitution sooner than the other. If you have sent an order to the Wine Merchant at Henley he will not be hurt at your countermanding it, as I understand you had made his acquaintance when with Mr. Joyce.[7] By the way, was Mr. Joyce ever paid for your last visit of tuition, if not, can you tell me how long you were there, & how this matter must be settled.

I am sorry you have not been more regularly supplied with the provincial Papers — They disappear soon after their arrival & it is difficult to get them again — You will have one or two by this Post. Grove was taken in Monmouthshire & I sent him to Gaol. A more harden'd or obstinate young Fellow I never met with. He might have been liberated on bail if he would have confess'd, but I could not get a word to the purpose out of him. The trials will be interesting & I hope you will be there under the wing of a *Magistrate*.[8] You will be perfectly correct in calling on all the Gentlemen you name to me & I must add Dr. Bourne[9] to your list. I hope you are making additions to your acquaintance; but be sure to select such as are respectable "a man is known by the company he keeps" was there ever a truer saying? I shall be in solitude here till the end of next week, when your Sister will return.

My very dear Robert   Your affectionate Father

E. Jenner

You must consult Mr. Jenner as a Friend respecting your becoming a Candidate for the Demiship[10] — It would be a good thing — but remember interest *alone* will never obtain it — you must *read hard*.

1. See Letters 64, 71, 75, 78, and 97.

2. A London banker. See Letter 3, n. 7.

3. Robert lived to a ripe old age as a bachelor colonel in the army.   — Fisk, *Doctor Jenner,* p. 110.

4. John Kidd (1775–1851), M.D. Oxford in 1804. In 1822 he became Regius Professor of Physic.

5. Sir Christopher Pegge (1765–1822), M.D. Oxford in 1792 and Regius Professor of Physic in 1801. He and Dr. Robert Bourne (see n. 9, below) were the leading physicians at Oxford.

6. Martin Wall (1747–1824), M.D. Oxford in 1777.

7. The Reverend J. Joyce of Henley, with whom Robert had lived and studied before going to Exeter College. See Letters 64 and 71.

8. Jenner is referring to his own role as magistrate, or justice of the peace. See Letter 60, n. 2, and Letter 97.

9. Robert Bourne (1761–1829), M.D. Oxford in 1787.

10. Mr. Jenner's identity is not known, but he must have been considered a useful source of information about applying for a scholarship at Oxford. A demy, the recipient of a demiship, received half the allowance of a fellow.

78. To R. F. Jenner, Esq., Exeter College, Oxford, 2 March 1816

My dear Robert[1]

Your last Letter reliev'd me from an anxiety I naturally felt respecting your health, for you express'd yourself more vaguely in your Letter than in your quotation, as in the former nothing was said about your having taken a Cold, but that you were unwell; so I was left to guess at the nature of your indisposition. I trust you have attended to my suggestions with regard to the Wine, & that you have only sent for a sufficiency for present use. You will be coming home ere long & we can talk more about this *poisonous* business when we meet. You know my fixt & unalterable opinion of Wine, as far as regards its deleterious effects on the human constitution.

Catherine,[2] who is writing at the other end of the Table, says you owe her a Letter & have been long her Debtor.

The Papers inform you what a ferment the House of Commons is got into — You will see by the Glostr. Herald that our County has call'd a Meeting for this day, consequently I do not yet know the result. Mr. Cassel (Brother of the Mayor of Bristol) who shot Ld. De Clifford's Game Keeper has *bolted*. The Keeper who was with Cassel, is taken & committed. Nothing new has come out respecting the Poachers — They affect to consider the Matter lightly. Sergt. Best, I understand is engaged as their Counsel. I do not see how they are to get off for if they be aquitted on the first Count (the Murder) how are they to escape from the second — the taking an illegal Oath?[3]

George is still disengaged from the Nuptial Knot — J. & Car: are still on their visit at the Davies's.[4]

Two of your late Letters were missent thro' careless superscriptions.

Your affectionate Father

Edwd. Jenner

Berkeley
Sat: night   March 2 1816

[*On the back in another hand, probably Catherine's:*][5] After spending a pleasant week at Chavenage with Harriet & Miss Sheppard — This is all the news I have to tell you — Have you heard any thing of the Marsleys. It would be a good thing if you could call on them I think. We heard from J. Vigel the other day. He was very well when he wrote which was in September. We had a long walk to Stone[6] & back yesterday & call'd on all the Stone People.

Wm. Davies & his Wife came here on Thursday to have the Infants vaccinated. I return'd from Kingscote last Monday.

1. See Letters 64, 71, 75, 77, and 97. The first paragraph was published in Jacobs, "Edward Jenner," p. 752.
2. Jenner's daughter.
3. The *Gloucester Journal* of 22 January 1816 reported on the murder of William Ingram, Lord Berkeley's gamekeeper, by poachers. Complete details of the trial, which led to the execution of two men, were reported on 15 April 1816. Jenner, as magistrate, had to participate in the trial at Gloucester, where he stayed at John Baron's house.   — Baron, *Life,* 2:221–22 with further comments by Jenner, pp. 415–16. See also Fisk, *Doctor Jenner,* pp. 264–65.
4. The Reverend William Davies, Jenner's nephew, lived nearby at Rockhampton. See Letter 93.
5. She also addressed the letter.
6. About three miles from Berkeley.

79.   To Doctor Charles Parry, M.D., Gay Street, Bath, 31 August 1816

Berkeley 31 August 1816

Sadly, most sadly, disappointed! I had carv'd out an excursion, my dear Charles,[1] which promised me many gratifications, but all hopes of their being realiz'd are gone among the Gas. I am fasten'd to this place by a chain so massy that it is quite impossible for me to move. No inconvenience of consequence, with regard to *the Ceremony,*[2] I trust will arise out of this disappointment. I am aware that there are other ceremonies ramifying from the parent stock & if you would have the kindness to see that they are amply executed, the obligation shall be properly acknowledged when I come to Bath for I by no means think my visit is put off for any length of time.

With regard to Pathology. The impression at present on my mind is that somehow or another the Milk of the Mother is capable of receiving impregnations which affect the Child. We have not yet made out *all* the odd things going forward in the animal economy. Tell me how it comes to pass that if I drink a glass of good Cider my Urine smells as fragrant as the bottle when just uncork'd? I don't give this as a paralel [*sic*] case, but as a puzzle. There must be a short cut from the Stomach to the Bladder. Shall we ask Riddle about these things? What if we were to fill the Stomach of a Puppy with Mercury, first tying up the Intestine, & then give it a good squeeze?

Pray tell your good Father I have got his Letter & shall write largely to him ere long — I most richly deserve his reproaches.

My best wishes to Mrs. P. & the young Ladies —
Ever Yours   My dear Friend

Edwd. Jenner

1. Charles Henry Parry, the son of Jenner's old friend Dr. Caleb Hillier Parry. See Letter 17, n. 6, and also Letters 80, 81, 90, and 91. The second paragraph was published in Jacobs, "Edward Jenner," pp. 752–53 and in Miller, "Letters," p. 16.

2. Augusta Bertie Parry was Jenner's goddaughter, and this probably refers to her christening. See Letter 80.

80.   To Dr. Charles Parry, Gay Street, Bath, 15 October 1816

Chauntry Cottage[1]   Berkeley
Oct: 15 — 1816

My dear Charles[2]

I am happy in writing to you, & making, *for me,* rather a quick reply to you last Letter. The beauty of my God-daughter[3] must be secur'd at all points & I have sent her the enclos'd little present to guard her from the spells of the Fiend that takes delight in spoiling Ladys' faces. Mr. Norman had better use the points[4] on the arms of some Cottage Children, & having produc'd a Pustule (Vesicle if it must be so) to vaccinate from that. I mention this because the Lymph fresh from the Arm is more certain than when inspissated, even (as per experiment) tho' it has not been dried five minutes. Emma[5] I think had but one Pustule, which I fancy went thro' its course undisturb'd — However, it would do the Lady no harm to *test* her from her Sister's arm. The matter sent is fresh from as fine a Pustule, as ever was call'd up by Vaccine Lancet. Some Dolts, Walker of Oxford & Kin[g]lake of Taunton, have lately been writing some alarming Stuff in the Yellow Journal[6] declaring thro' thick & thin that all the V. Matter now in use is worn out by being work'd so long. Pretty analogy this — "the world is young." Now the fact is, that this par nobile had got some that was ruin'd from contamination by some individual whose skin (from disease) was incapable of producing that which was correct. This sort of decompos'd rubbish, I am sorry to say, gets into the hands of the ignorant & produces local disgrace. "The world is in its infancy."

The question is, respecting the Stomach in the Nursery, whether that is in fault, or whether Mrs. Parry's milk is in a state fit to meet its powers of digestion? I should think the latter & to put the thing to issue, I would have you give the little one a meal or two, from a new milk-pail. The substitutes for milk I believe are all bad. The best deviation I have found from the maternal milk is that of the Ass — the next is the Cow's diluted with one third part of water, with a very small portion of Sugar. But not unfrequently the process of Vaccination acts like a charm in correcting deviation in the abs[o]rbent System, & you know it is a doctrine in my School, that the Stomach is the first — the root, the foundation, the Governor of the whole family. Away with the term Scrophula — Let us have something expressive of morbid action, or disease of the Lymphatics. You know how long I have been an Hydatid-Hunter[7] & tho' Time has brought me to a hobble, yet I scramble after my Game as hard as I can. And what do you think? I seem to see him now popping out of a Lymphatic. A speck, or specks, (small hydatids) appear where a like portion of the Lymphatic is lost. "The World's a Baby."

I don't take in the Institution Journal,[8] but both the others; I must see this paper on the Metals, because you say 'tis good. How goes on Geology? I think I have made out something about the Pebbles in our Basaltic-amydaloid Rock. I wish you would look at your Oolite thro' a good magnifyer. I find — (stop — I fancy so) they are made up of concentric layers; the first cry[s]taliz'd on a small atom, a fragment of stone. You really should see, with a geological eye, the Country around this place — the diversity it presents would delight you. And if my good old Friend[9] in the Circus would but accompany you, then after a day's hunt we would sing old Rose & burn the Bellows. I really want to sing a Swan-like Ditty to him before — — — I want too, to write to him; but when I think of setting about it my head seems so full, I know not how & so it is put off till tomorrow, tomorrow & tomorrow. "The world's a Foetus." Adieu my dear Charles — Bob & Catherine[10] desire their best affections with myself to you, Mrs. Parry & the accomplish'd Miss Emma.

Most truly Yours

Edwd. Jenner

PS. No Cheltenham for me, this winter —

1. The name of Jenner's house. With fifteen rooms, it was certainly an oversized cottage.

2. See Letters 79, 81, 90, and 91. From the advice given here, Jenner evidently served as the Parrys' physician. This letter was published in its entirety in Jacobs, "Edward Jenner," pp. 753–55, and the discussion in the second paragraph on hydatids was published in Miller, "Letters," p. 16.

3. Augusta Bertie Parry. See the inscription Jenner wrote in a Bible he sent her in Baron, *Life,* 2:295.

4. Quills, metallic instruments, or ivory blades which were used to collect and distribute vaccine matter. Jenner eventually decided that ivory was preferable.

5. Parry's older daughter.

6. Richard Walker, Esq., of Oxford and Robert Kinglake, M.D. Glasgow in 1794, of Taunton frequently published in the *London Medical and Physical Journal.* There is an article by Walker "On the Analogy between Natural Small-Pox, Inoculation, and Vaccination" in the

October and November 1815 issues (34:295–301, 387–93) and also one "On the present State of Vaccination in Oxford" in the February 1816 issue (35:93–98).

7. For a review of Jenner's various comments on hydatids see LeFanu, pp. 98–100. There are many observations on hydatids in F. Dawtrey Drewitt, ed., *The Note-Book of Edward Jenner in the Possession of the Royal College of Physicians of London* (London: Oxford University Press, 1931).

8. Probably the *Journal of Science and the Arts,* edited at the Royal Institution of Great Britain, 1816, vol. 1, which contains on pp. 126–31 an article by A. B. Granville entitled "A Report on a Memoir of Mons. Methuon, entitled 'Découverte de la Manière dont se forment les Cristaux terreux et metalliques non salins, &c.' Read before the Geological Society, the 16th of February, 1816."

9. Dr. Caleb Hillier Parry, the father of Charles.

10. Jenner's son and daughter.

81. To [Dr. Charles Parry], 22 February 1817

Berkeley
Saturday 22nd Feb: 1817

My dear Doctor[1]

Having just heard that a neighbour of mine is setting off for Bath, I avail myself of the opportunity of making an inquiry for your poor Father.[2] I consider the time long since I last heard, & beg you give me a line soon. — Remember me most kindly to him.

Bakewell[3] call'd upon me yesterday in his way to Bristol, where he is going to give a Course of Lectures, if he can get hearers. Do beat up for him, if you can enlist any scientifics, it will be good for both Parties — My best affections at both your Houses.

Truly Yours

Edw. Jenner

1. Although unaddressed, this letter was undoubtedly written to Charles Parry. See Letters 79, 80, 90, and 91.

2. Caleb Hillier Parry. In October 1816 he had suffered a stroke from which he became paralyzed on the right side and had speech impairment. See Letters, 1, 14, 17, and 57.

3. Robert Bakewell (1768–1843), geologist. "From 1811 onwards he lectured on geology all over the country, exhibiting sections of rock formation and a geological map, the first then of its kind." — *DNB.*

82. To John Ward, Esq., Ryeford near Stroud, 16 July 1817

My dear Sir[1]

Mr. Fletcher[2] has thrown you into a tremendous storm, & while that is pelting you pray don't think of coming to Berkeley. However, this I mention by way of precaution only, not as a prohibition, as I shall certainly be at all times happy to see you. As matters have undergone so great a change since I last saw you, Mr. F. from an inspection was certainly better able to determine the nature of the malady than myself, without an inspection, & I trust his decision is correct — then all will be right again.

You have sent me a very fine specimen of the arsenical Pyrites for which I am much obliged to you; but as nothing is more interesting to me than organic Remains, especially Bones, I hope you will bear in remembrance your promise respecting those in possession of your Father.

If you should be prevented coming, pray write & believe me with best wishes

Yours very truly

Edwd. Jenner

Berkeley
16th July 1817

1. John Ward cannot be identified. He was probably a patient and friend of the family. See also Letter 86.

2. Possibly William Henry Fletcher (d. 1853), "for many years Surgeon to the Gloucester Infirmary" and at one time surgeon to Gloucestershire Yeomanry Cavalry.   — Plarr's *Lives of the Fellows of the Royal College of Surgeons of England*, 2 vols. (London: Royal College of Surgeons, 1930), 1:406. Stroud is in Gloucestershire.

83.   To the Reverend Richard Worthington, Swindon Villa, Cheltenham, 26 January 1818

Berkeley Jan: 26 1818

You speak to me, my dear Doctor,[1] about indulging hope. I have almost done with this business, & 'tis very odd one should continue to grasp at it so long, when 'tis as slippery as a soap'd Pig's tail. Did you ever watch little Boys running after Butterflies? A pretty picture of Hope this. And now about *Corporal Strength* & animal Spirits. The Corporal is in tolerably good condition & fit for service; but of the latter, if I give any account at all, it must be such a miserable one, that I will spare the feelings of a Friend, & say nothing.

What you heard of Robert's[2] sleeping two or three nights at Cheltenham was not true. He dozed away I understand one forenoon there. Young Men of Spirit, well train'd in the *blood red Hunt* must not sleep o'nights. This would be natural, consequently tame & insipid. One found guilty of anything so weak & so much in the common order of things, would be banish'd the Society, unless it was under the Table & it could be first prov'd that he had at least three bottles in his Stomach. Robert has not yet taken a plunge into the Castle Pandaemonium; but I fear he sometimes gets within the sulphurated atmosphere.

What; poor Maria not well yet? The Fashionable remedy is Laurel leaves, made limp by the Fire like the leaves of the Cabbage, when used as an application. As for myself, I have not a fair chance, as I am toss'd about in Carriages from morning till night over roads, I should suppose as bad, as ever the Coachman of Julius Cesar drove over. You little think what a condition this Swindon-battered Shoulder of mine is in — seldom free from pain by day, & at night it often so terrifies poor quiet Morpheus, he won't come near me. What is all this about Beavan & the Blues?

I must not forget to tell you that I have a weekly stock of Vaccine fluid, some of which shall become solid & cross the Atlantic whenever you will order it. A Letter at the same time might be useful, as the Matter (which I shall take care to mention) has not been many months taken from its original source; and all they have now in use, in America, has been passing there from arm to arm for nearly the fifth part of a Century.

Catherine[3] is still on the Hills — at the ill-fated House of Kingscote where she officiates as first nurse. I begin to think the burnt girl[4] will recover — poor, dear Harriet's case remains undetermin'd. I shall never prevail on any one to keep a Shower Bath in some corner of a Nursery; charg'd. Were a Child on fire, it might be extinguish'd in an instant, & indeed just as soon on a full grown female. Well — such a Letter as this for length has not been thrown off the nib of my pen for many a month. Shall you be ever able to get thro' it? Certainly not, if I go on much longer; so adieu my good Doctor & with kind regards to all at the Albion,[5] believe me most sincerely Yours

Edw. Jenner

1. See Letter 67, n.1. This entire letter, with the exception of the second paragraph about Jenner's son Robert, was published in Baron, *Life,* 2:417–18; the fourth paragraph was published in Miller, "Letters," p. 16.

2. Jenner's son Robert, at this time twenty-one.

3. Jenner's daughter.

4. Probably Caroline Marienne Kingscote, the niece of Jenner's wife. She is mentioned in Jenner's letter to the Reverend W. Davies (Baron, *Life,* 2:416–17), where the nursery fire is also mentioned. Her older sister, Harriet Frances, was buried at Kingscote in May 1818. — "Pedigree of Kingscote, of Kingscote, in Gloucestershire," in Thomas Dudley Fosbroke, *Berkeley Manuscripts* (London: John Nichols and Son, 1821), facing p. 218.

5. One of the Cheltenham hotels.

84. To Dr. Edward Jones, Montgomeryshire, 7 April 1818

Berkeley April 7 1818

My dear Sir[1]

The very pleasant & interesting correspondence that took place between us some years since, have not escaped my recollection. Your early exertions in the cause of Vaccination I trust were not of public utility only, but that you have reap'd many private advantages from them. Accept my best thanks for your present communication on this subject. There is not a civiliz'd spot on any part of the Globe where the practice is not now very generally adopted.

Your Letter dated the 5th reach'd me this evening, the 7th which is as soon as it could come. I shall write by this post to Cheltenham, but am fearful that my Letter will not arrive till Thursday evening which may not be quite so soon as the Montgomery party. At this season of the year Lodgings of every description are easy to be procured, from the Cottage to the Mansion. It is probable that ere long I may make an excursion there for a few days. Should this be the case, I shall have great pleasure in paying my respects to the Ladies & offering my assistance in any way in my power.

Believe me, dear Sir,   with great respect   most sincerely Yours

Edwd. Jenner

1. See Letters 19, 24, and 30. Jones had obviously written to acquaint Jenner with Montgomeryshire relatives or friends who were coming to stay at Cheltenham.

85. To Miss Mary Dyer, Dawlish, 16 August 1819

Berkeley
Aug: 16, 1819

My dear Mary[1]

Before I say one word to your Mamma in reply to her kind Letter, I must turn my attention to your nice *Folio.* This ought to have been done long ago & certainly would have been, but since this tropical heat has enveloped me, I really have been fit for nothing — neither for working nor thinking; yet my brain is not so completely codled in this atmospheric caldron as to render me quite insensible to your kindness in indulging me with so long a Letter, and I may add, (had it not been for one or two crooked sentences) so pleasant a one. The *window scene,* for example, after the hot Bath was not quite as one could wish. But was that the fault of the Gentleman with the *Latin* name, or your's? I cannot for a moment suspect Mamma's want of vigilence.

When some Friend of the family — was it not Major Adey? — named a Gentleman at Dawlish as a medical prodigy, I had not the least notion it was one with whom in earlier days I had a good deal of intercourse, & of a kind far more unpleasant for him than for me; tho' not pleasant to either — but tell me when my name was mention'd to him how he relish'd it? This mystery shall be unravell'd one of these days. Perhaps you may think I know no more about you & the party, than what your Letters communicate. If you think so, you must forget some of the propensities of your native Town,[2] where it has been my fate to be dragg'd three or four times a week for some time past, & it is at some of these excursions that I *read* the Dawlish Gazette. Before the little accident happen'd to your Father, a Paragraph asserted "that so gay was the Wotton party at Dawlish that Mr. Sam Dyer was going to give a Ball." I will not fill up my Letter by further quotations. I knew of your intended stay till October, perhaps before you had quite made up your minds to the new arrangement yourselves. Charming Wotton! Well, this is harmless kind of prattle, & so is that which takes place now & then, as I ambulate your Garden at Combe, between me & old William.[3] The sombre walk there between the two high green walls is well calculated for contemplation, and there I should indulge but William is too proud of his Stocks (now blossoming a second time), his Celery, & the immensity of his Onions, to suffer me to remain long unmolested. The Garden, I must say, is as much attended to, as if its cultivator had a superintendant.

What Mr. D. says of Plymouth & Dock makes one long to behold these stupendous works of Nature & of Art combin'd[4] — The Son of my Friend Mr. Dunning[5] grew better & I hope continues so; & this event has suspended my Journey. I shall expect to see the Cabinets of the *Geologist* much improv'd by the Dawlish Fossils on her return — Has she found any bones among the blue Lias?[6] Bid her look sharp — and pray what is Miss Jenny about? Has some kind green wave been good enough to compress her lip to its due thickness? My Love to both & best regards to all.

After the pleasing intelligence your Mamma has given me, there is no room for a moment's hesitation respecting your prolonging your stay — and I should say to the utmost period conveniency will permit. As for Miss W — — let her dash & splash as long as she likes. Is she such an Idiot as to put Fashion in competition with health. Such nonsense is not to be listen'd to a moment. The Sea is doing you all a great deal of good — it is a kind

Friend — & on this kind Friend you are entreated to turn your backs & shew ingratitude — Fie Miss Webb! Is this a part of the moral system you inculcate? Adieu my dear Mary & believe me with best affections

Most sincerely Yours

Edw. Jenner

P.S. How fortunate it was for Mr. Dyer to have so able & immediate an attendant as Mr. Sam when he met with the accident. Let me hear again soon.

1. Although unidentified, Mary Dyer was obviously the daughter of a family friend who was vacationing at Dawlish, a seaside resort on the Devonshire coast south of Exeter. In the account of Jenner's funeral in the *Gloucester Journal,* 10 February 1823, a Mr. Dyer, Esq., was in procession with the corpse.

2. Wotten-under-Edge, a town not far from Berkeley, where Jenner had attended school as a child.

3. Probably the Dyers' gardener.

4. Jenner may be alluding to the mile-long breakwater designed by John Rennie, on which construction had begun in 1812.

5. Richard Dunning, a Plymouth surgeon. See Letter 63, n.3.

6. A blue limestone rock found in southwestern England.

86. To J. Ward, Esq., [Autumn 1820]

My dear Ward[1]

I am very sorry to find that Miss Worthington is ill — Your account of it was the first that reach'd this place. She is in good hands; hands that will doubtless be exerted in cuffing the aerial Monster Influenza till he takes flight or sinks into — from whence he came. I did hope in the course of nearly three months, the period of my illness, I should have had the benefit of the *hands* I allude to; especially as I recd. what was considered by me as a promise from time to time. Since I saw you, I have made scarcely any progress towards recovery; but on the contrary rather made the retrograde motion. I purpose taking a little Carriage exercise tomorrow — the first time for the period I have named. Writing is painful to me, & on this acct. you will excuse this scrap — the Seat of my Malady is now in my head. The dreadful Tale from Weymouth reach'd me from Fry, three or four days ago. I hope it may save some of our young Folk here from drowning, which has been near happening two or three summers past.

Adieu — Truly Yours

E Jenner

I have sent the Flute.

Dialogue
Well — Peer or not; I think this Duke
Deserves a pretty sharp rebuke.
— Why what a Ninny are you Dan, —
A Duke's above a Gentleman.

1. See Letter 82. The following note in another hand is on the reverse of the letter:
"of Vaccine celebrity — The epigram is also by Dr. J. and was elicited by some slight on the part of the Duke of Beaufort towards a company of Gentlemen who had met to dine together on a political occasion. I believe his Grace was expected & sent an excuse which was not thought to be satisfactory

"Dr. Jenner died of Apoplexy Jan. 26 1823 after having had several warnings, one of which is alluded to within. This letter was written in the Summer of 1819."

There is no evidence that Jenner had a serious illness in the summer of 1819. More probably this letter dates from the autumn of 1820, following the 6 August 1820 attack which he suffered while walking in his garden. It is described in Baron, *Life*, 2:308–10.

87. To Dr. Forrester, Derby, 9 February 1821

Circular[1]

Berkeley Feby. 9
1821

Dear Sir

[*two-page printed circular*]

very truly
Edw. Jenner

[*Note on blank page 3:*]

Dr. Jenner hopes his Friend Dr. Forester will excuse the formality with which he is address'd in the *Circular,* and when convenient, favor him with an answer.

Not being acquainted with any of the Surgeons in Derby, he had no alternative but that of writing to Dr. Forester, tho' probably he himself has not practic'd Vaccination.[2]

1. This is a four-page leaflet of which pages 1 and 2 bear a printed text (LeFanu 96). During the smallpox epidemic of 1816–19, many fell ill who had previously been vaccinated. Jenner republished at Gloucester in 1819 his article "On the Varieties and Modifications of the Vaccine Pustule Occasioned by an Herpetic State of the Skin" (LeFanu 82), which had first appeared in 1804. Two years later he distributed this circular letter in which he asked colleagues to send him their experiences on the effect that skin diseases had on vaccination.

2. This implies that it was customary for only surgeons to perform vaccination.

88. To James Johnson, Esq., Governor of the Corporation of the Poor, St. Peters Hospital, Bristol, [1821]

Dr. Jenner presents his Comps. to Mr. Johnson & has sent him a Copy of his Circular,[1] not with any expectation of his returning an answer to his Queries, but merely to shew him that he is again endeavoring to point out the *Rock* to the Faculty on which so many of them have split, either thro' ignorance or heedlessness. He will see that Dr. Jr. pointed out its position many years ago. He was much pleas'd to observe, from an advertisement brought to him by Mr. Langharne,[2] that Mr. Johnson is still persevering in his endeavors to save the suffering Poor from the Fangs of the Smallpox which lately made such lamentable havoc in the City of Bristol.

1. See Letter 87, n. 1. Although a small, rectangular clipping from another piece of stationery bearing "28th 1819" in another hand is pasted on the back of this letter, there is no evidence whatever that Jenner was distributing a circular then. The date could be no earlier than 1821.
2. Langharne seems to have operated a delivery service between Berkeley and Bristol. He is also mentioned in Baron, *Life,* 2:424.

89. To Miss Elizabeth Pruen, Dursley, 26 August 1821

My dear Miss Eliz:[1]

Pray tell me how it comes to pass, that I have neither seen or heard anything of Mr. T. Pruen since his return from Guernsey?

The Animal you have sent me is a beautiful specimen of the Lizard of the Country. Tho' you sent him in a condition so relax'd & languid, he has already got into very good spirits.

Pray tell your Sister how good & how kind I thought it of her to write me a Letter while she was *abroad;* so amusing & so instructive. When I have the pleasure of seeing her, she will I trust go on with the History of her Travels.

With best wishes to the Family, very truly Yours

E Jenner

PS. All alone — Catherine at Bath — Robert at Sidmouth — Susan — Caroline & their aunt at Burbage.[2]

Sat. Night 26 Aug: 1821

1. The daughter of Jenner's friend Thomas Pruen. See Letter 54.

104

2. Susan and Caroline were twin daughters of Jenner's grandnephew, William Henry Jenner. They were descended from Jenner's brother, the Reverend Henry Jenner of Burbage.

90. To Dr. Charles Parry, Circus, Bath, 14 September 1821

N.B.   The following down to mark // was written before I received your last Letter.

My dear Friend[1]

A few days since, I think 'twas Tuesday, I received from Nicholls[2] a Proof of the intended Pamphlet on Factitious Eruptions[3] — By return of Post I sent to request he would print off another, & send it to you; & perhaps ere now you have received it. How different a thing is a Manuscript & a printed Copy — In the latter those blemishes which are in great measure eclipsed by the former become prominent. Fosbroke[4] had the manuscript to dress up before it went to the Press; but I don't much like the *Fashion of his Cut* here & there. The first sentence is quite unintelligible, but that admits of easy arrangement. The Notes which form some of the most interesting parts of the Work might perhaps be incorporated with it, with advantage to its general appearance; but on this point I had rather that others decided than myself.

I see but little prospect before me at present of my visiting Elmhurst, tho' it certainly would afford me great pleasure to pay my respects to the interesting family there. Respecting Bath, I cannot of course say anything now — No intelligence has reach'd me since your last account.

You have probably seen my Daughter ere this — She will of course soon return, having paid a long visit to her Friends. My Nerves are not quite so susceptible of the *sharp* noises as they have been, but still I feel myself unfit to venture among those who do not thoroughly know my unfortunate habits. Could I but call the wooden Spoon & Trencher into use again at our Tables; and instead of a Glass, the Maple Bowl — (Oh Dear, 'tis soothing to think of it) how smooth the tide of life would glide along.[5]

//

All this, my dear Friend, was written before I received your last Letter. I know not what to do with the Proofs — You and I think alike about the Style of what flow'd, or rather dash'd off, from the pen of our young Professor. Time, & an absence from his father's[6] Study, will lead him into more sober paths — At present he gets too much into the Zig-zag. He is coming here tomorrow I find in his way to Bath. You will find him docile & good temper'd; and I think his being with you a few months will produce mutual advantages. I have not yet received your corrected Copy; but I have a dread about me at the idea of publishing it; at least till it has undergone considerable changes. And yet I shall vex at seeing it go into the Fire; for it contains a good thing or two. Could not some of those terrible long notes in which are involv'd much of the best part of the performance, be interwoven with the text? But 'tis a shame for me to plague you so much about it who have at present so many cares & solicitudes of your own.

Best wishes   Faithfully Yours, my dear Friend

E Jenner

14 Septr. 1821

1. See Letters 79, 80, 81, and 91.

2. John Nichols, a London printer. See Letter 92.

3. This was a preliminary printing of LeFanu 109, *A Letter to Charles Henry Parry, M.D., F.R.S. &c &c, on the Influence of Artificial Eruptions* . . . (London, 1822), of which a copy dated 1821 exists in the Edinburgh University Library (LeFanu 109a). See LeFanu's discussion (p. 86) of the extensive revision of this version, of which 500 copies were mistakenly printed.

4. John Fosbroke had been Jenner's assistant at Cheltenham. He was the son of the Reverend Thomas Dudley Fosbroke and received the M.D. degree from the University of Edinburgh in 1830. He published a chapter on Jenner in Thomas Dudley Fosbroke's *A picturesque and topographical account of Cheltenham and its Vicinity* . . . (Cheltenham: S. C. Harper, 1826), pp. 271–300.

5. For Jenner's increasing sensitivity to sharp sounds, see also Letter 95.

6. Jenner's old friend the Reverend Thomas Dudley Fosbroke, who published "Biographical Anecdotes of Edward Jenner" in his *Berkeley Manuscripts* (London: John Nichols, 1821), pp. 219–42.

91.   To Dr. Charles Parry, Circus, Bath, 10 December 1821

My dear Doctor [1]

I have been a little alarm'd by an advertisement that appear'd in one of the Bath Papers, & by another on the Cover of the Gentleman's Magazine, announcing the Publication of *the Book*. [2] On looking it over attentively with some friends after Fosbroke's departure for Edinburgh, Errors were discover'd that would have made it perfectly ridiculous — However by cancelling two or three of the Sheets I am in hopes it will after all its misfortunes come out in a state that may be worthy your inspection. Another fortnight I hope, may strew these, like other autumnal leaves, over our Vallies. Little did I think there would have been such a piece of work about so small a matter.

I have not been entirely inattentive to the *Rocks* — several specimens are put up — But I must stop from further research for the present, as most of them are got into their old quarters; a state of submersion.

How is Mr. Bedford & all the Family in the *Clouds*? All right I hope in the Crescent.[3] Best wishes — most truly Yours

Edw. Jenner

The Chauntry
10 Decr. 1821

1. See Letters 79, 80, 81, and 90.
2. See Letter 90 for a discussion of the difficulties surrounding the publication of Jenner's last book, caused by the ineptitude of his editorial assistant, John Fosbroke.
3. Corrected, in another hand, to "Circus."

92. To Messrs. Nichols, 25 Parliament Street, London, 1 February 1822

Berkeley   Glostershire
Sir[1]   Feb: 1 1822

I am happy to find that the printing of the Pamphlet[2] is at length accomplish'd & should be obliged to you to send by the usual conveyance (the Gloucester Coach) 25 Copies directed for me at Berkeley. The London List shall be sent in a few days — will you be kind enough to slip a Note into the Parcel to say whether my direction respecting the distribution shall be sent to Mr. Baldwin[3] or to you?

I remain   Your obedient & faithful Humble Servant

Edw. Jenner

1. John Nichols and Son, the printer of Jenner's *A Letter to Charles Henry Parry . . . on the Influence of Artificial Eruptions* (London, 1822) (LeFanu 109).
2. See Letters 90 and 91.
3. The bookseller. The book was printed by Nichols for Baldwin, Cradock, and Joy, Paternoster Row.

93. To the Reverend Dr. William Davies, F.A.S., 9 February 1822

Dear William[1]

I can hardly make my mind up to suppose that in so short a space of time as the Note within specifies, I have beclad my sides with four new Coats!

Have the goodness to shew it to one of your Brothers[2] & if he should think I have been so extravagent, let the account be settled out of my means. They will know something about this business as they settled my last account with the Baron, & perhaps can refer.

Yours truly

Edw. Jenner

9th Feb: 1822

1. The Reverend Dr. William Davies, curate of Rockhampton, Jenner's nephew. His father, also named William (1741–1817), was the husband of Jenner's sister Anne, and was vicar of Eastington. — Thomas Dudley Fosbroke, *Berkeley Manuscripts* (London: John Nichols, 1821), facing p. 220.

2. The Reverend Robert Davies, curate at Stonehouse, and Edward Davies, surgeon at Ebley. — Fisk, *Doctor Jenner,* p. 261.

94. To Charles Dumergue, Esq., Albemarle Street, 17 February 1822

My dear Sir

This will be deliver'd to you by my ingenious Friend the Rev: Robert Ferryman[1] — a gentleman who was intimately acquainted with your late Uncle, from whom he received many marks of kind attention.

I hope you & your Family are well —

With best wishes   very truly Yours

Edw: Jenner

1. See Letter 64, n. 2.

95. To Dr. Alexander J. G. Marcet, 14 Harley Street, London, 5 March 1822

My dear Friend[1]

Allow me to thank you, which I do most heartily, for your kind Letter & pressing Invitation to visit you at your Villa.[2] How delightful this would be, were it practicable for I believe the man does not exist who has a truer relish for scenes such as you enjoy, than myself. But alas! my dear Marcet, this cannot be. My health since last we met, & made the pleasant excursion to visit our valued Friend at Enfield[3] has suffer'd considerably. I do not know that any of the ordinary machinery belonging to life has yet suffer'd materially; but this I know that the most important of all vital Organs, the

Brain, does not perform its offices with that smoothness & regularity as it was wont to do. The deviation I have chiefly to complain of, is a morbid sensibility to sharp sounds, so that I am really debar'd from going into any society beyond the circle of my own family, for it requires a constant attention on their parts to prevent the ordinary noises occasion'd by the use of common domestic utensils — such as Knives, Forks, Spoons & such like striking against Cups & Saucers, Plates &c. It is not every sound that affects me alike — To some I am far more indifferent than to others — What might be term'd a *hollow sound* makes but little impression, such as the ringing of a Church Bell — a Man hooping a Barrel, or hallooing; but it is the *sharp* sounds emanating chiefly, as I have mention'd, from the utensils which spread over our Tables at breakfast & dinner which annoy my Nerves in this distressing way. In a Female I should call it Hysterical — but in myself I know not what to call it, but by the old sweeping term nervous. Will you allow me to call it electrical? No matter what name it may bear — if you can point out any mode of alleviation, I know you will — I have hitherto made but few attempts on a supposition that these symptoms do not arise from mere morbid determination of blood to the brain, but that there must be something mechanically wrong.

Your Friend Herberski,[4] who brought me your dispatches, was good enough to spend two or three days with me. He has plenty of intelligence about him but still thirsting after more — all this is quite right. His Fellow traveller, Holst[5] from Norway, I found also an intelligent Man. Either of these Gentlemen could have imparted much instruction on the subject of Vaccination, I am almost sorry to say, to many of our Practitioners here. You must recollect, tho' it is no[w] seventeen years ago, my imparting to you the importance of our selecting for the purpose of Vaccination those Childre[n] whose skins were free from Eruptions part[icularly] those which bear the Herpetic Character.

//

Four months at least have elapsed since I wrote the above, & tho' you will call this a queerish kind of an incident, yet I rejoice at its having happen'd, as I trust it will completely do away your *piano* charge of having forgotten an old Friend. No, my dear Marcett, my Brain must lose many many a slice more of intellectuality before it can forget you. I rejoice exceedingly at your being once more amongst us — for now you are on this side the channel I feel, as it were, in contact with you; & believe me I am happy in the enjoyment of that feeling. What is become of Herberski? I shew'd him all the attention in my power & gave him on his departure a large packet of

Letters &c &c for delivery on his return; but I have heard nothing of him since; nor has any individual to whom I address'd my Circular[6] ever taken the least notice of it. I want to say a thousand things to you — but can only add my kindest & best regards to you & my amiable Friend Mrs. Marcet. You shall hear again soon.

Edw: Jenner

Berkeley
Chantry Cottage   March 5 1822

1. See Letter 7, n. 1, for the complete list of the twenty-two letters to Marcet in this collection. Jenner must have forgotten Marcet's medical degree, for he addressed the letter to "A. Marcett Esqr." The square brackets occurring in three places indicate holes in the paper. Jenner's comments about his health were published in Miller, "Letters," p. 17.

2. Marcet's villa in Switzerland. In 1819 Marcet had retired from the staff of Guy's Hospital and had returned to Geneva to live. He returned to Britain in the fall of 1821 to spend the winter in London. The following summer he visited Scotland, and in the fall, while passing through London on the journey back to Switzerland, he was "attacked with gout in the stomach" and died in Great Coram Street on 19 October 1822.   — DNB; London Medical & Physical Journal 49 (1823): 85–88, where his death date is given as 18 October.

3. Dr. William Saunders, who had retired to Enfield in 1814 and died in 1817. This June 1814 visit was arranged in Letter 72.

4. Possibly Vincent Vladislav Herberski, M.D. Vilna 1812, who was adjunct professor with Joseph Frank in the Vilna Clinic from 1813 to 1824, and then professor of special pathology and therapy until his death in 1826.   — August Hirsch, Biographisches Lexikon der hervorragenden Aerzte aller Zeiten und Völker, 6 vols. (Vienna, 1884–88), 3:176.

5. Frederik Holst (1791–1871), M.D. Copenhagen 1817, was appointed Christiana city physician in 1818 and spent 1819–22 traveling to Denmark, Germany, France, England, and Ireland to study the medical care of the poor and insane. He eventually became one of the leading physicians in Norway.   — Hirsch, Biographisches Lexikon, 3:282–83.

6. See Letters 87 and 88.

96. To the Reverend William Pruen, Fladbury near Evesham, 14 June 1822

My dear Sir[1]

I never make any one a promise without an intention of fulfilling it. That which I long since made to you respecting my begging your acceptance of some utensil that had long been in my service has not escaped my memory; and finding that your Brother is going to Fladbury tomorrow, I avail myself of the opportunity of sending you what I think you will not dislike; the very pen, which under my guidance has travell'd over many an unexplored region; & which under the self same guide, is this moment in motion.

How goes on Vaccination? I feel under obligations to every one who pursues it with even half the ardor & attention that you do. Without the latter, the former may defeat even well meant intentions. When you fall in with any of the neighbouring Faculty, convince them if you can of the vast importance of attending to the state of the skin when they vaccinate. You have my Circular[2] I think on this important subject; but lest you should not, I shall send you another copy. Perhaps you may think it too much of an interference with the medical profession if you try the effects of the plan I have suggested for stopping the progress of disease by means of the artificial Eruptions;[3] but if that be the case, you may possibly be able now & then to rouse the attention of your medical acquaintances.

Make my best wishes to Mrs. Pruen and your family, and believe me Most truly Your's

Edwd. Jenner

Chantry Cottage
June 14 1822

1. This is probably the brother of Jenner's close friend, the Reverend Thomas Pruen. See Letter 54, n.1.
2. See Letters 87 and 88.
3. Jenner is alluding to the information contained in his *Letter to Charles Henry Parry . . . on the Influence of Artificial Eruptions* (London, 1822).

97. To Robert F. Jenner, Esq., Cheltenham, [date unknown]

Dear Robert[1]

I sent for Giles yesterday while Dr. Davies was here. He (Giles) was much surpris'd at hearing that the Dog which the Boys brought into the Field where Knight was, had been represented by Ormond as a *Lurcher,* as it was in fact nothing more than a *Bull Terrier,* a dog as likely to catch a Comet as a Hare — Without going into detail, I need only say that the *Doctor* is not only willing, but desirous of signing the proper Document for the liberation of James Knight but I presume it must have your signature also. Giles said he knew nothing reproachable in Knight's character, altho' as I understand, Ormond said he would give him a bad character were he at the Sessions.

Be as quick as you can, in what you do in this business.
Your affectionate Father

Edwd. Jenner

Berkeley
Wednesday Morning

1. See Letters 64, 71, 75, 77, and 78. Robert had become a magistrate assisting his father. — Fisk, *Doctor Jenner,* p. 264.

98. To the Reverend George Jenner, in his absence to Miss Jenner, [date unknown]

Monday Night

Dear George[1]

I should be obliged to you to request the favor of Mr. Joyner to fill up the entries in my Tax paper as before with this exception, that I have now only one Man servant; — one Horse only I believe was enter'd in the last Paper & I have the same now. I have given notice at the Office here that my entrys are made at Berkeley.

I hope you will feel no more Headaches —

Truly Yours

Edwd. Jenner

You can easily sign my name to the Paper.

1. Jenner's nephew. See Letters 27 and 99. Jenner's statement about having only one manservant and one horse suggests that the letter was written towards the end of his life after his daughter's marriage in August 1822.

99. To the Reverend G. C. Jenner, Stone [date unknown]

Dear George[1]

Capital — I hope you have got some young Trees fit for transplanting. There is some fine Fruit in my own Garden — I pick'd a Goosberry this morning which weigh'd five Drachms full weight — I shall send it to you if I can get a Box — but it loses weight rapidly by keeping.

I saw the poor Woman this morning — she looks & is quieter than she was — Being out of office my powers are diminish'd — I will do all I can for her.

Could she not be got into St. Lukes? There is a good deal of form in the business, but she would be judiciously treated here.

Truly Yours

Edw. Jenner

PS   I shall think Stone[2] will be as hard as its name, if it does not think of you properly for the benefits you have conferr'd.

1. See Letters 27 and 98.

2. The village three miles south of Berkeley where George had finally secured a living in the church.

100. To C. F. Hausserman, Esq., Ebley near Stroud, [date unknown]

My dear Sir[1]

After so long an acquaintance you must have discover'd that I am a very impatient sort of a Gentleman. You will not be surpris'd therefore at my soliciting you to furnish me as speedily as you can, with the Ebley Case of *Tic Doulereaux.* I hope this may find you at home & that you will take up a bit of paper & give me a reply with as much speed as you can. Even as far as it went, until the unfortunate interference of Dr. D — — was quite enough to convince me of the power of *the Pustule* in regulating some of those movements of the Brain which are deranged & assume a wrong action.[2]

I never hear anything of Mr. Cross, which is vexatious. A Pamphlet is order'd for him from Town, and if you see Mr. Jones, tell him I shall send him one the first opportunity.

Great news today from Ebley House — It[3] seems to have had a good effect on poor Edward, as he reports himself better. I hope he will steadily persevere in a plan of diet that will prove duly nutritious without heating the Brain.

With best wishes   Yours my dear Sir   very truly

Edw. Jenner

1. Although Hausserman's identity has not been discovered, this letter leads one to speculate that he was a local surgeon.

2. This idea was developed in Jenner's pamphlet, *A Letter to Charles Henry Parry . . . on the Influence of Artificial Eruptions* (London, 1822). See Letter 90, n. 3, and Letter 96.

3. A marginal note in another hand reads: "Tartar emetick applied exterior."

101. To an unknown man, [date unknown]

My dear Sir[1]

I thank you for your Letters of yesterday & today; the former gives a clear detail of the late occurrences in our sick room; but still no light arises to direct us to form a correct judgement of the case. As I said before, the *Delirium* was in my opinion hysterical & the piercing pain of the Head is probably a link of the same chain. In a late unfortunate case, I saw too much of this. It was sometimes confined to a spot, characterizing the Clavus Hystericus,[2] but not unfrequently it would occupy a considerable portion of the Head. Leeches, or the single puncture of a Lancet, always afforded relief. My hopes rather increase with the late accounts you have given than otherwise — but as I shall see you soon I will suspend further observations till we meet. This should be tomorrow did not an engagement interfere & prevent my coming till the day following; Friday we will then have a full conference.

Yours my dear Sir   Most truly

Edw. Jenner

Berkeley
Wednesday Night   April 1st

1. This letter, showing Jenner functioning as a medical consultant, is obviously directed to a medical colleague.

2. The medical terminology for the sensation which feels as if a nail were being driven into the head.

102.   To Thomas Pruen, Esq., [date unknown]

To T. Pruen Esqr.[1]

Let the usual Puncture be made in the arm with a Lancet — then introduce the coated extremity of the Ivory Point, & suffer it to remain near a minute, supporting it in its place by the gentle pressure of the finger, when the oozing fluids will dissolve the concreted vaccine Virus & the Patient be probably infected. I say *probably,* because the dried vaccine matter tho' quite fresh, like that I consign to you, sometimes fails to infect while that which is taken in its fluid state in some early stage of the Pustule & inserted immediately from arm to arm, does not disappoint me once in five hundred times.[2]

E J

1. Jenner's close friend. See Letter 54, n. 1. This is actually not a letter, but rather, Jenner's instruction to Pruen on the correct method of vaccinating. Undated, it was written sometime after 1802 and before 1812, when Pruen acquired a living in the church and was thereafter addressed as the Reverend Thomas Pruen. Preserving the virus on an ivory point is not advocated in Jenner's printed *Instructions for Vaccine Inoculation,* which appeared between November 1801 and February 1802 (LeFanu 60).

2. In Letter 80 Jenner suggested to Charles Parry that the point which he had sent for the vaccination of his goddaughter should first be used on "the arms of some Cottage Children" to produce a pustule from which Parry's daughter should then be vaccinated.

APPENDIX

OTHER DOCUMENTS CONCERNING THE EARLY HISTORY OF VACCINATION

A-1.   David Ramsay to Henry Laurens, Jr., 3 June 1794

Charleston   June 3d 1794

Dear Sir[1]

Your favor of May 28 was this day reviewed together with the seven canal scripts.[2] These shall be exchanged for the new ones as soon as they are ready.

I send you inclosed variolous matter on glass.[3] I inoculated two people from it & both have taken. It should be moistened with a drop of cold water & then introduced on the point of a lancet or sharp stick.

Mr. Warner has given in his estimate to Mr. Smith. I am glad to hear you will so soon be in town. Hoping you have found Mrs. Laurens & daughter well & that they & you are returned safe to Mepkin.[4]

I am affectionately yours

David Ramsay[5]

1. Henry Laurens, Jr. (1763–1821), was the brother-in-law of David Ramsay.   — *David Ramsay, 1749–1815: Selections from His Writings,* ed. Robert L. Brunhouse, *Transactions of the American Philosophical Society,* n.s. 55, pt. 4 (1965): 26. This letter was published as no. 216.

2. Scrip: "A preliminary certificate . . . issued after the allotment, usually on payment of the first installment, to one who has subscribed for stock of a bank, railroad, or other company. . . . When all installments are paid, the scrip is exchanged for a bond or share certificate." — *Webster's New International Dictionary.* Ramsay was president of the stockholders of the Santee Canal Company.

3. The live smallpox virus used for smallpox inoculation, the preventive measure which had been adopted in Britain and her colonies in the 1720's and was widely used by the end of the century. Edward Jenner's substitution of cowpox as the inoculated substance a few years later initiated modern vaccination against smallpox. The context of this letter addressed to a layman shows that variolation, or smallpox inoculation, was performed by nonmedical people. In this instance perhaps Laurens intended to inoculate his slaves.

4. The name of Laurens' estate.

5. David Ramsay (1749–1815), a graduate of Princeton and the medical department of the College of Philadelphia, had settled in Charleston, S.C., in 1773 and become one of its

leading citizens. His numerous publications, chiefly on history, include *A Review of the Improvements, Progress, and State of Medicine in the 18th Century, Delivered January 1, 1801* (Charleston, 1801). See also Letters A-2 and A-8.

A-2. David Ramsay to Dr. White, Waynesborough, Georgia, 22 July 1802

Charleston   July 22d 1802

Sir,[1]

Your obliging favor of May 24th arrived safe. Like you, we have few cases of vaccination[2] among us at present. The small pox have disappeard & the dread of that disorder drives many to inoculation either old or new. Besides most who chose vaccination have received it. The credit of it is stronger than ever. I scarcely know any persons of consequence who are unbelievers in Vaccination. Charleston has abounded with cases of the natural small pox following the inoculated small pox one of which provd fatal. This with its circumstances has satisfied the most timid that there is at least as much safety in the new as the old inoculation. The case was too important to pass without notice. I therefore gave a paragraph to the Times printer about it which you will find under the Charleston head under a seperate to lessen the expence of postage.[3] The more public this case is made the better for the community. Their interest in the progress of vaccination is great. Physicians are the only persons who will lose by that capital discovery.

Dr. Rush of Philada. has lately sent me a few copies of Jenner's instructions for vaccination reprinted in Philada.[4] I have also got the same from Dr. Waterhouse in Boston.[5] I inclose you one on the genuineness of which you may rely.

We have annexed vaccination to our new dispensary in this city. An address in favor of vaccination as contrasted with small pox inoculation to the patients of the dispensary is also inclosed.[6] The day of doubt is over. I believe there will be very few persons hereafter inoculated for the small pox & that vaccination will spread triumphantly round the world. No spurious case has yet happened among us. Where the least doubt existed a second vaccination was ordered. If men undertake to vaccinate who have no knowledge of medicine they may bring a temporary cloud on the business; but great is truth & will prevail.

We are remarkably healthy. Only twelve whites have died in Charleston in the first 20 days of this month. No [*hole in paper*] fever. An epidemic catarrhal complaint has been general but it yields to medicine. Mr. Floyd of your place was inoculated for the small pox & resisted it. This I had also printed in the Newspapers. I am with   great respect   Your most obedient Servant

David Ramsay.[7]

1. Joshua Elder White (1775–1820), a Pennsylvania native educated in Georgetown, D.C., had married a Georgia woman and was practicing in Waynesboro. In 1802 he made a topographic, meteorologic, and epidemiological survey of Waynesboro and vicinity, the first systematic account of disease in Georgia, which was published in the *New York Medical Repository* in 1806. After moving to Savannah in 1804 he eventually abandoned medicine for business. In 1816 he published the travel book *Letters on England: comprising descriptive scenes; with remarks on the state of society, domestic economy, habits of the people, and condition of the manufacturing classes generally,* 2 vols. (Philadelphia: M. Carey, 1816).   — Victor H. Bassett, "Two Physicians and Two Periods in the Medical History of Georgia," *Journal of the Medical Association of Georgia* 29 (March 1940): 137–42.

This letter was published as no. 258 in Brunhouse's edition of Ramsay's letters (see Letter A-1, note).

2. An early use of the word *vaccination,* which had been coined by Jenner's friend Richard Dunning of Plymouth and introduced in his *Some observations on vaccination* (London: Cadell and Davies, 1800). The more common expression for a number of years was *vaccine inoculation.*

3. The following account appeared, without signature, in the 19 July 1802 issue of the *Charleston Times:*

"Died, on the 9th instant, in the 6th year of her age, of the small-pox taken in the natural way, Miss *Leah Cardoza,* daughter of Mr. David Cardoza. She had been inoculated for the small-pox some years before, and was supposed by all concerned to have then had that disease.

"Since last January, six or seven other cases have occurred in this city, of persons taking the small-pox in the natural way, after having been, in the opinion of physicians and others, successfully inoculated for it. It is remarkable, that of several hundreds who have been vaccinated in Charleston, nothing of the kind has happened, for in no instance has the small-pox followed the vaccine disease. In Mr. Cardoza's family, his infant son Aaron was vaccinated several weeks ago, and by the sole aid of this vicarious disease, he has hitherto escaped the small-pox, though exposed to it by constantly associating with his lately deceased sister, through the whole period of her last illness, till her death; and even sleeping in the same bed with her after her small-pox had broke and run. Twelve days have now elapsed since the decease of Miss Leah, in which period, infection (if any had been received) would certainly have shewn itself in her surviving vaccinated brother Aaron; but he continues to enjoy uninterrupted health, and furnishes a convincing proof of the complete security the vaccine disease affords against the small-pox."

The 16 July 1802 issue of the *Times* contained an article, reprinted from the *Boston Centinel,* in which Benjamin Waterhouse disproved alleged small-pox cases following vaccination. He also reprinted a letter from Edward Jenner and stated that although it had not been longer than five months since he sent vaccine matter to Charleston, the latter had already established vaccine institutions for the poor, undoubtedly referring to the Charleston Dispensary (see n. 6, below).

4. Dr. Benjamin Rush had been Ramsay's teacher in Philadelphia. LeFanu does not mention a Philadelphia reprint of Jenner's *Instructions*. See the following note.

5. *Extract of a letter from Dr. Jenner, dated London, February 24, 1802. Instructions for Vaccine Inoculation* (LeFanu 61). The letter was addressed to Waterhouse, the first American promoter of vaccination. No place of publication is given; either it was reprinted in both Boston and Philadelphia, or Waterhouse had sent Rush copies for distribution which Ramsay mistakenly thought had been reprinted in Philadelphia.

6. The Charleston Dispensary had been created by the Medical Society in 1801. The title of the address was *The Physicians of the Charleston Dispensary to the Patients of that Institution* (Charleston, 3 May 1802). —Joseph Ioor Waring, *A History of Medicine in South Carolina, 1670–1825* (Charleston: South Carolina Medical Association, 1964), pp. 136, 146.

7. See the previous letter, n. 5.

A-3. John Coakley Lettsom's Proposal for the Jennerian Fund, [1802]

To commemorate illustrious actions, has been the glory of civilized nations — Rome decreed a civic crown to him who saved one citizen; what then is due to Dr. Jenner, whose discovery of Vaccine Inoculation, has already saved the lives of millions of fellow creatures, and which by its general extension may extirpate the most fatal and lothsome disease that ever desolated the earth; and, which has destroyed every year by accurate calculation five hundred thousand infants in Europe alone! This great discovery has astonished mankind, not less in magnitude and utility, than by the urbanity of its author, in communicating to the world, a secret, by which he might have acquired incalculable wealth; but elevated above every sordid consideration he gratuitously conferred an inestimable blessing on his fellow creatures, and taught them to preserve their helpless offspring from the ravages of the smallpox.

The British Parliament, after the most careful investigation, hailed him the sole Discoverer of this efficacious Preservative; and under this impression, at the conclusion even of an expensive war, unanimously acknowledged it, by voting a gratuity, expressive of the national obligation.

The zeal that actuated Dr. Jenner, to promote the knowledge of his Discovery, so interesting to the whole human race, led him to expences almost commensurate with the liberality of Parliament. — A Discovery so wonderful and so unexpected, at first, rather dazzled than convinced mankind, of its infinite importance — even to many scientific men, it appeared almost incredible. They humanely indeed wished to see realized what they deemed impossible — Time at length, and the most decided experience, have established forever, providentially for the human race, this salutory Discovery, and a grateful community, anxious to commemorate an Epoch, so auspicious to human existence — a Discovery of which the Records of history afford no adequate comparison, propose to announce a subscription to raise a fund for the purpose hereafter explained, and invite the co-operation of the Friends of Humanity, not only in Great Britain, which boasts the birth of Jenner, but in every part of the world; for every portion of it, is interested in this godlike Discovery, which has for its objects, *The preservation of Human existence, and the general felicity of the human race.*

1. A Committee shall be appointed in London, to receive subscriptions from, and to correspond with every part of the world.
2. The amount of the subscriptions shall be considered as a public property, to be invested in the Funds, in the name of Trustees, and to be called THE JENNERIAN FUND.
3. The principal of which shall remain for ever, as a memorial of the Discovery of Vaccine Inoculation by Dr. Jenner.
4. The annual interest shall be devoted to Dr. Jenner and after his death, to his right Heirs, descendible as a fee simple for ever.
5. In default of Heirs, three of the oldest persons of the name of Jenner, then living in England, shall be found, who shall draw Lots, under the direction of the Trustees, and the one whom fortune shall favour, shall succeed to the receipt of the interest, and become a new stock of inheritance; and, in case of a second failure, the same method shall be pursued, and so toties quoties.[1]

Early in June 1802 the House of Commons had voted to award Jenner £10,000 for the discovery and propagation of vaccination. This was thought insufficient by many colleagues, among them Thomas Beddoes, Sir Gilbert Blane, and John Coakley Lettsom. Lettsom (1744–1815) was a prominent London physician, famous for his philanthropy, who in 1775 had attempted unsuccessfully to extend smallpox inoculation among the poor. He became a staunch supporter of Jenner and helped to organize the Royal Jennerian Society. Lettsom wrote to Jenner as follows: "I was truly chagrined on seeing the niggardly reward voted by the House; and had double that sum been asked, it would have been granted: however, as an individual, I am not disposed to stop here; but immediately to set on foot a subscription that should invite every potentate and person in Europe, America, and Asia, because every avenue of the globe has received, or may receive, your life-preserving discovery. This subscription should not be for you, but it should be a fund the interest of which should be for ever devoted to the name of Jenner." — Baron, *Life*, 1:517–18. This proposal was superseded by the second Parliamentary grant of £20,000 awarded in July 1807.

1. The British custom of honoring a hero's name forever is still preserved today in the descent of titles. The ninth Lord Nelson, the modern descendant of the first Lord Nelson of Trafalgar fame, is a police sergeant in Hertfordshire.

A-4. John Coakley Lettsom to C. Perkins, Esq., Camberwell, 7 December 1805

To C. Perkins Esq.[1]

Not having received the favour of an answer to my letter of Nov. 29th last, I imagine that in consequence of personal application to Mayo, the fact has been satisfactorily ascertained, that he never had the least vestige of the Cow-pock;[*] at the same time, I cannot but return thanks to my young friend, for his candour in informing me, of the suspicion he entertained of the fallacy of the Cow-pock, as a security against the small pox. Had every opponent of vaccination acted with equal candour, the illusion by which credulous, and alas! unfortunate parents have been misled, and the consequent deaths of thousands of their children would have been prevented, as well as all those lothsome afflictions, which the small pox often excite in the constitution. I have now under observation, a young woman, who will be lame through life, and two children, in whom the small pox pustules have pushed an eye of each youth out of the sockets; and one of the children is blind in both eyes, with a face so disfigured, as scarcely to resemble the human.

About 60,000 persons who have been vaccinated, have since been inoculated with the smallpox, without a single instance of the latter having been produced. About 3 years ago, some children of the Foundling hospital were inoculated with the Cowpock and for the sake of experiment (which however is now totally unnecessary, as a person is known to remain unsusceptible of the small pox, after having really had the Cowpock) they have been recently inoculated with the smallpox, without any one of these having taken this disease. I enclose the account communicated by Dr. Stanger,[2] as well as Dr. Dundas' relation of a fatal case of inoculation of the small pox under the direction of Dr. Moseley;[3] and Lord Egremont's letter on the success of vaccination at Petworth for perusal.[4]

Happily for the human race, in consequence of the unequivocal success of the Cowpock, and the dreadful mortality of the smallpox (within the last week, making 168 hours, no fewer than 113 children have been killed in London alone, by the smallpox), many institutions have been lately formed for exterminating the latter, the following facts being now established, by

---

[*]This has been confirmed by Beane, Forbes, and Aveline, the three respectable surgeons of the village.

the experience of Europe, Asia and America — two physicians only, in Europe, excepted, as I have before observed.

1. That the cowpock is a security against taking the smallpox.
2. That the cowpock is never fatal; nor does it produce more subsequent disease or humours, than drinking the milk of the cow.

    Whilst in another view,

3. That the small pox kills about 50,000 British European subjects annually, every one of whom might have been saved by the cowpock.
4. That inoculation of the small pox is frequently fatal, and at all periods has encreased the mortality of the smallpox.

These facts have induced me against the pecuniary interests of my own profession, from principles of humanity, patriotism, and conscience, to endeavour to exterminate the smallpox, which can be alone effectually done by vaccination in the opinion his friend

John Coakley Lettsom [5]

London Dec. 7, 1805

PS. As the happiness of the Community is deeply interested in the subject of different inoculations, I propose, with your kind permission, to print our letters in the next edition of my expositions,[6] not as a party matter, but for the sake of suffering humanity; if however my young friend, should not wish his name to appear, it certainly shall be omitted.

1. Unidentified, but probably a local surgeon.

2. Christopher Stanger (1759–1834), M.D. Edinburgh, was physician to the Foundling Hospital in London. He tried unsuccessfully to make it possible for all qualified physicians in London to become Fellows of the College of Physicians.

3. Benjamin Moseley (1742–1819), physician to Chelsea Hospital, was a "violent opponent" of vaccination, publishing a great number of articles and books against it.

4. Sir George O'Brien Wyndham, third Earl of Egremont (1751–1837), patron of the arts, was a leading figure in London. At Petworth House in Sussex, one of his estates, he had created a college of agriculture. In February 1800 Jenner demonstrated the efficacy of vaccination by personally carrying out the procedure on nearly 200 persons at Petworth. — *DNB*, 21:1159–61; Baron, *Life*, 1:369.

5. For Lettsom, see unnumbered note to Letter A-3.

6. Lettsom is referring to *Expositions on the Inoculation of the Small Pox, and of the Cow Pock* which he had first published anonymously in July 1805, and reissued under his name in the beginning of 1806. Although the second edition contains much new information and excerpts from some of Lettsom's correspondence, it does not contain Perkins' letter.

A-5. Sir George Thomas Staunton to — — —, 20 February 1806

Canton   Feby. 20th 1806

My Dear Sir

I had the pleasure of receiving your letter of the 13th of March last per favour of Mr. Annandale, and wish it had been in my power during his stay in China, to have shewn him more effectually the esteem I entertain for your recommendation.

The busy scene in which we are engaged here for a few months in the year by the lading and despatch of a numerous Fleet of Merchantmen, affords few if any topics, which are worthy of communication, or deserving your attention, and I assure you I look forward with anxiety to the day on which I may be able to extricate myself from all concerns of this nature, in order to return to a much better Country and rejoin the pleasing and instructive Society in which I have so often had the pleasure of meeting you. — [1]

It will not be uninteresting to you to hear that we have at length introduced into China Dr. Jenner's valuable discovery of the Vaccine inoculation, and that altho' the virus was obtained from Manilla by the assistance of the Spaniards,[2] yet the Surgeon of the British Factory Mr. Pearson[3] has the merit of pretty considerably dispersing, and I hope permanently establishing the practice, in this populous Capital — It would have proved difficult to have so quickly overcome the objections and scruples of the Chinese against every kind of innovation, if Mr. Pearson had not hit upon the plan of writing a concise treatise on the discovery & mode of operation,[4] which by the assistance of a native Chinese following the Medical profession I had the honor to translate into the Language of this Country. The Work has been published & gratuitously distributed at the expence of the Company,[5] and as it is novel & unique in its kind I take the liberty of enclosing you a copy. —

I have written to my cousin B. A. Brodie whom you probably see often, and therefore I need say nothing in remembrance

I beg to subscribe myself   My Dear Sir   with sincere regard & esteem   Your most faithful Servant

Geo. Tho. Staunton

1. Sir George Thomas Staunton (1781–1859), who wrote extensively on China and knew the language well, had traveled to China as page with his father, Sir George Leonard Staunton, in 1792. In 1798 he was employed by the East India Company as a writer in its Canton factory. He was promoted to supercargo in 1804 and to chief in 1816. After returning

to England in 1817, he served in the House of Commons for many years. In 1823 he helped to found the Royal Asiatic Society.

At this time age twenty-five, Staunton did not return to England for eleven more years.

2. The vaccine had been brought to Macao in the spring of 1805 by a Portuguese merchant of Macao. It was carried on live subjects from Manila, who had been vaccinated with virus brought by Francisco Xavier de Balmis on the royally sponsored Spanish expedition to eradicate smallpox throughout its overseas possessions. After some Macao vaccinations by Portuguese practitioners and Alexander Pearson, senior surgeon of the East India Company, the virus was lost. It was reintroduced by Balmis himself on 10 September 1805, with three Filipino children as carriers. — Alexander Pearson, "Respecting the Introduction of the Practice of Vaccine Inoculation into China A.D., 1805: Its Progress Since that Period, and Its Actual State," Report submitted to the Board of the National Vaccine Establishment, dated Canton 18 February 1816, *Chinese Repository* 2 (May 1833): 35 ff. See also Michael M. Smith, The *"Real Expedicion Maritima de la Vacuna" in New Spain and Guatemala, Transactions of the American Philosophical Society*, n.s. 64, pt. 1 (1974): 59. For an extensive account of the history of smallpox inoculation and vaccination in China, see K. Chimin Wong and Wu Lien-Teh, *History of Chinese Medicine,* 2nd ed. (Shanghai, 1936; facsimile, 1973), pp. 273–301.

3. Alexander Pearson, whose report was cited in the previous note, was formerly a resident of Liverpool, had served as surgeon on the *Arniston* from 1795 to 1803, and had become a member of the Royal College of Surgeons in 1801. In February 1805 he joined the East India Company in Canton as surgeon "but not allowed to engage in private trade." In the same year he acquired a St. Andrews medical degree. Retiring in 1831, he died in London on 25 December 1836. — D. G. Crawford, *Roll of the Indian Medical Service, 1615–1930* (London, 1930), p. 624.

4. Jenner's friend Thomas Pruen wrote in his *Comparative sketch of the effects of variolous and vaccine inoculation, being an enumeration of facts not generally known . . .* (Cheltenham, 1807), pp. 40–41, as follows: "At the request of Mr. Drummond, the Chief Supercargo at Canton, Mr. Pearson, a medical man there, drew up an account of Dr. Jenner's discovery." This suggests that the idea for the book was Drummond's and not Pearson's.

5. The East India Company. The book was also sponsored by a Hong merchant, "it being indispensable that Books printed in China should appear the production or be sanctioned by some Native holding a public situation." — Wong and Wu, *History of Chinese Medicine,* p. 278. The original printing of 200 copies was soon used up, and according to Pruen, writing in 1807, three editions were issued, the third of which added the account of the Balmis expedition. In 1828 Staunton published *Miscellaneous notices relating to China, and our commercial intercourse with that country,* pt. 2, for private circulation only (Havant: I. Skelton, printer), containing "Abstract of the contents of a Chinese treatise upon vaccination, by Alexander Pearson, translated into Chinese by G. T. Staunton" with the note: "The abstract on Vaccine inoculation at end, is printed in Chinese characters on double leaves, printed on one side only." See Baron, *Life,* 2:82–85, 356, for other letters concerning the Staunton translation.

A-6.   Sir Henry P. S. Mildmay to [John Coakley Lettsom], 28 January [1808]

Sir

I can have no objection to accept the Honor of becoming one of the Vice

Presidents of the Jennerian Society, & you will be pleas'd to signify the same to the Committee.

I cannot but avail myself of the opportunity to express my very earnest wish that some Report may be publish'd to the World as soon as possible respecting the unfortunate occurrences which have lately happen'd at Ringwood.[1] It is quite necessary that the Committee should be aware that they have, in some measure, shaken the faith of this part of the Country in the efficacy of Dr. Jenner's discovery: and therefore, the sooner, & the more generally that the Report of the Committee is circulated, the better. If there has been any mismanagement with respect to the Persons vaccinated, I trust, that no false delicacy will prevent the Committee from exposing it, as the failures at Ringwood are much dwelt on by the Enemies of our Institution.

I understand also that there is another instance of a Child of Dr. Harness of the Transport Board, who is said to have taken the small Pox after vaccination, which ought to be investigated.

I am persuaded that the Committee will forgive me for mentioning these particulars, which I do from no other motive than an anxious desire to have every possible cavil remov'd from the efficacy of a discovery which I consciously believe to be the most important & valuable of modern times.

I have the Honor to be   Sir   Your most obedient   very humble Servant

H P S Mildmay[2]

Dagmersfield Park
Jany. 28 [1808]

1. In September 1807 smallpox appeared at Ringwood in Hampshire. Although vaccination was initiated the following month, a number of vaccinated individuals contracted the disease, an event which fueled the antivaccinists' cause and led to numerous articles in newspapers and periodicals. — Baron, *Life,* 2:108–10. See also Letter A-7.

2. Sir Henry Paulet St. John, 3 Baronet, who assumed the surname of Mildmay on 8 December 1790, was born in 1764 and died on 11 November 1808. His obituary in the *Gentleman's Magazine* (78, pt. 2 [1808]: 1045) reads as follows: "Nov. 11. At Bath in his 44th year, Sir Henry Paulett St. John Mildmay, bart. M.P. for Hampshire. His complaint was a diseased liver with which he had been afflicted for many years, and endured the suffering of a long illness with manly firmness and patient resignation. Sir Henry generally resided at Dagmersfield park, near Odiham, and lived in a style truly magnificent. His hospitality, like his manners, was liberal and open; and, from his general condescension to his inferiors, and his munificent donations to the poor, he is sincerely lamented. He has left a wife and fifteen children." A letter from Mildmay to Jenner is published in Baron, *Life,* 1:590–91. This letter was probably, but without proof, addressed to John Coakley Lettsom, who played a major role in the Royal Jennerian Society.

A-7. William Blair to Okey Belfour, Esq., Royal College of Surgeons, 29 January 1808

To Okey Belfour Esqr. — Secy.

Sir,[1]

I feel it my duty, as a member of the College, to request that you will lay before the Board of Curators a new anonymous Publication; which, I am told, has been announced to the common people, by large posting-bills on the walls of this Metropolis! It is entitled, *"The fatal Effects of Cowpox Protection" &c at Ringwood;* and, you will see that the author (who is one of the Court of Assistants)[2] has not only traduced the Royal College of Physicians therein, but fraudulently printed some of the private papers, known to be in the custody of the Curators! I beg also to inform you, that the same author has very recently insulted the College by another anonymous publication, resembling a Newspaper, called *"The Cowpox Chronicle;"* of which the Chairman (Mr. Long)[3] has a copy, & I have shewn it to Mr. Cline.[4]

I am ready, Sir, to explain more of his insidious & truly unprofessional conduct, in the Ringwood affair, when required; though I have already told a few particulars to different worthy & respectable Gentlemen of the Board.

The honour of our Royal Colleges & the good of the public, so shamefully treated, will justify me in thus formally addressing our Board of Curators.[5]

I am, Sir, Your humble & obedient Servant

W Blair[6]

29th Jany. 1808
Gt. Russel Street, Bloomsbury Square

1. Okey Belfour was the secretary of the Royal College of Surgeons.

2. The author was John Birch (1745?–1815), surgeon to St. Thomas's Hospital and Surgeon extraordinary to the Prince Regent. His epitaph reads, "The practice of cow-pocking, which first became general in his day, undaunted by the overwhelming influence of power and prejudice, and by the voice of nations, he uniformly and until death perseveringly opposed, conscientiously believing it to be a public infatuation, fraught with peril of the most mischievous consequence to mankind." — *DNB*.

As a consequence of Birch's attack, the Royal Jennerian Society appointed a medical investigating committee, composed of John Ring, William Blair, and Dr. J. S. Knowles, who went to Ringwood and carried on two days of investigations. Their report, favorable to vaccination, was published in the *Gentleman's Magazine* (78, pt. 1 [April 1808]: 344) and in the *New Annual Register* (London, 1809), March, 1808, pp. 45–46.

The Court of Assistants was part of the hierarchy of the Royal College of Surgeons.

3. William Long was on both the Court of Assistants and the Court of Examiners of the Royal College of Surgeons. — *A List of Members of the Royal College of Surgeons in London* (London, 1805), pp. 3, 4.

4. Henry Cline (1750–1827) was surgeon of St. Thomas's Hospital and a lecturer on anatomy.

5. Blair eventually published the Ringwood material in *Hints for the Consideration of Parliament, in a Letter to Dr. Jenner, on the supposed Failure of Vaccination at Ringwood; on the prevalent Abuse of variolous Inoculation, and on the Practice of the Smallpox Hospital* (London, 1808).

6. William Blair (1766–1822) was director of the Royal Jennerian Society. See also Letters 44 and 45.

A-8. David Ramsay to Dr. L. Myers, Georgetown, 16 February 1808

Charleston Feby 16th 1808

Dear Sir,[1]

I have this day received your favor of the 12th instant & I shall by the next mail send you vaccine fluid inclosed in this letter taken as late as may be not to lose the post.

I think that the fluid is best & most easily taken & preserved & transmitted on the point of a quill. I now use that mode exclusively. All old & dry preparations of it are uncertain especially in warm climates & persons. They may do for a few days but the older they are the greater is the risque of their failing. I have proceeded with dry matter brought 800 miles & 17 days old but there were but a few successful cases out of many attempts. The durability of the vaccine fluid though true in cold countries does not hold to a great extent in Charleston. I once succeeded only in one case of vaccination out of 26 when the matter was old. From the moment the fluid is perceptible I begin to use it & I think the earlier it is taken the better though as long as it remains fluid it may do sometimes.

I have made no recent experiments for testing the vaccine by inoculating for the Small Pox. It is as fully ascertained that the vaccine preserves from the small pox as that the inoculated small pox preserves from the natural.

The report of the committee of physicians on the efficacy of the vaccine appointed by authority in England[2] ought to satisfy every body. They collected information from all public institutions for vaccination & from hundreds of private practitioners all over England. The report was an unanimous opinion that Vaccination afforded perfect security against the small pox: In consequence of this report the Government of England has lately given to Dr. Jenner £20,000 in addition to their original grant of £10,000.[3] These who beleive [*sic*] that all the physicians in England are fools & that the Government of that country gives away large sums of money for nothing may doubt of the efficacy of vaccination, but to all rational men the point is as satisfactorily proved as that the Peruvian bark cures intermitting fever.

The eruptions which we find to follow the Vaccination are rare. I have seem them as often to follow the inoculated small pox as vaccination. Children with or without either are liable to many cutaneous diseases especially in warm climates. I am with great regard & esteem yours

David Ramsay[4]

After making an incision with the lancet I introduce the point of the quill. Both quills are armed at the point.[5]

DR

1. Dr. Myers has not been identified.

2. *Report of the Royal College of Physicians of London on Vaccination. With an Appendix, containing the Opinions of the Royal Colleges of Physicians of Edinburgh and Dublin; and of the Royal Colleges of Surgeons of London, of Dublin, and of Edinburgh* (London, 1807).

3. See Letter 21, n. 3.

4. On Ramsay, see Letter A-1. This letter was published in *David Ramsay, 1749–1815: Selections from His Writings,* ed. Robert L. Brunhouse, *Transactions of the American Philosophical Society,* n.s., vol. 55, pt. 4 (1965), no. 279.

5. Meaning that they have been coated with vaccine matter at the point.

A-9.   Jean-Nicolas Corvisart to Henri-Marie Husson

A Monsieur
Monsieur Husson[1] Docteur en Médecine etc.
Rue des Maçons Sorbonne, la 3e. ou la 4e. porte cochère
   à gauche en montant

Si vous voulez, mon très cher Confrère, faire trouver votre enfant chez moi à deux heures précises, aujourd'hui, je m'en servirai pour vacciner l'enfant pour lequel je vous ai demandé etc.

Tout à vous

Corvisart[2]

ce mercredi 27

Un mot de réponse pour que je prévienne.

1. Henri-Marie Husson (1772–1853) was one of the early vaccinators in France, where vaccination was introduced cautiously but systematically. As lymph kept on threads deteriorated easily, doctors preferred to use lymph taken from the arm of a recently vaccinated child. In his monograph *Recherches historiques et médicales sur le vaccine* (Paris, 1801), pp. 29 f., Husson lists Corvisart among the early adepts of vaccination, together with Thouret, Hallé, Sabatier, Pinel, Guillotin, Andry, Jeanroy, and J. J. Leroux. See Robert G. Dumbar, "The Introduction of the Practice of Vaccination into Napoleonic France," *Bulletin of the History of Medicine* 10 (1941): 635–60. This letter was transcribed and annotated by the late Henry E. Sigerist. See Letters 11 and 66, above, addressed to Husson.

2. Jean-Nicolas Corvisart (1755–1821) was Napoleon's favorite physician.

A-10. Joseph-Ignace Guillotin to Henri-Marie Husson, Paris, 23 August 1808

A Monsieur
Monsieur Husson,[1] Secrétaire du Comité Central de Vacine
rue du Battoir — Paris —

Paris 23 aout 1808[2]

Je prie Monsieur Husson de vouloir bien donner du vaccin à Mr. Blozy, chirurgien, demeurant rue du Gros-Chenet, à Paris: je lui en serai très obligé.

J'ai l'honneur de le saluer

Guillotin[3]

1. See the preceding letter to Husson.
2. Below this, in another hand, possibly that of Husson: "Comité du 26 aout 1808."
3. Joseph-Ignace Guillotin (1738–1814), who suggested the use of the machine for the infliction of capital punishment named after him, was a prominent medical practitioner in Paris, member of the Constituent Assembly from 1789 to 1791. The Comité Central de Vaccination of which Husson was secretary in 1808 was constituted on 11 May 1800. This letter was transcribed and annotated by the late Henry E. Sigerist.

A-11. Embossed card signed by Oliver Houghton, Milton, Massachusetts, 25 October 1809

[*On the front of the card is a snake forming an ellipse. Above the snake:*]
Paper   He is slain   No 32

[Inside the snake:]
The twelve individuals whose names are written on
the back of this card were vaccinated by Doctr: Amos
Holbrook, at the town inoculation in July last; they were
tested, by Smallpox inoculation, on the 10th Instant, and
discharged this day, from the Hospital, after offering to the
world, in the presence of most respectable witnesses, who hono-
red Milton, with their presence on that occasion, an additional proof, of the never failing power, of that mild preventive
the Cow pock, against smallpox infection, a blessing great,
as it is singular in its Kind — whereby the hearts of men —
. . . Should be elevated in praise to the Almighty Giver
Oliver Houghton
Chairman of the Committee for
Vaccination [1]

[On the reverse, written in the ellipse:]
These twelve were the only individuals who expressed a desire
of being tested out of 337, vaccinated at the town inocul:
Joshua Briggs
Samuel Alden
Thomas Street Briggs
Benj: Church Briggs
Martin Briggs
George Briggs
Charles Briggs
John Smith
Catharine Bent
Sussana Bent
Ruth E: Horton
Mary Ann Belcher

1. In the summer of 1809, having been convinced that vaccination protected against
smallpox, the selectmen of the town of Milton, Massachusetts, undertook to hold a general
vaccination for the town's citizens. They hired Dr. Amos Holbrook to vaccinate on 20–22
July for twenty-five cents a person. More than a quarter of the citizens responded, leaving
fewer than twenty unprotected, since the remainder of the population had already been
immunized by previous exposure to smallpox. Milton was the first community in the United
States to arrange vaccination for its citizens. In order to reinforce the proof of the effec-
tiveness of vaccination, the twelve persons listed on the back of this card submitted
themselves to smallpox inoculation on 10 October. When they were discharged from the
hospital on 25 October, this testimonial card was issued.

The Milton town vaccination was imitated in other communities, and an unsuccessful effort was made to pass a state law requiring annual general vaccinations in each town. For a detailed account of the Milton experience and references to source materials see John B. Blake, *Public Health in the Town of Boston, 1630–1822* (Cambridge: Harvard University Press, 1959), pp. 183–88.

Amos Holbrook (1754–1842) had settled in Milton in 1777 and was given permission to operate an inoculation hospital there. He had a large practice in Milton, Dorchester, and Quincy. — C. H. Brock and Eric H. Christianson, "A Biographical Register of Men and Women from and Immigrants to Massachusetts between 1620 and 1800 Who Received Some Medical Training in Europe," *Medicine in Colonial Massachusetts, 1620–1820,* A Conference held 25 & 26 May 1978 by the Colonial Society of Massachusetts (Boston: The Colonial Society of Massachusetts, 1980), p. [130].

A-12. James Smith to David Shriver, Jr., Esq., Westminster, Md., 1 November 1810

Baltimore 1 Novr. 1810

Sir [1]

The managers being desireous [*sic*] to fix a day for the commencement of the drawing of the vaccine institution Lottery [2] as soon as the sale of Tickets might justify them to proceed with it wish to be informed of the progress you have made in disposing of the tickets left with you for sale. On this account be pleased to return or address to me on or before the first day of January next a list of the tickets left at your disposal, noting those which have been sold & delivered as well as any particular Ticket, or quantity of Tickets which may have been engaged, we will also thank you to inform us at the same time should any of the tickets left with you remain unsold, how many of them you have reason to believe can be disposed of for cash should we fix the time of drawing to commence at an early period.

The actual sales of tickets which have been already made and the numerous engagements entered into here to take tickets as soon as the drawing will be near at hand flatter us with a prospect that we shall be able to commence the drawing in the Spring . . . but of this you will be more particularly informed . . . in answer to your return of sales. . . .

Permit to inform you that the managers have fixed the rate of commission at three pr. cent and that this amount may be retained by any agent on all sales that he may have effected.

With Respect   Your Obliging Humble Servant

Jas. Smith

P.S.   Enclosed I send you a copy of the articles of an association which we are forming here & hope you may find it convenient to join it & also to obtain subscriptions for shares from any of your acquaintances who might be calculated on for punctuality in case any loss was sustained by the Company.

J.S.

1. David Shriver, Jr., has not been identified.

James Smith (1771–1841), a graduate of Dickinson College, Carlisle, Pa., had attended medical lectures at the University of Pennsylvania and been a disciple of Benjamin Rush. After settling in Baltimore he became a leader in public health. As founder and attending physician of the Baltimore General Dispensary, he began vaccinating on 1 May 1801 and the following March he opened a vaccine institution at his home, vaccinating the poor free of charge.   — Whitfield J. Bell, Jr., "Dr. James Smith and the Public Encouragement for Vaccination for Smallpox," *Annals of Medical History,* 3rd ser. 2 (1940): 500–517.

This letter is written in stylized script, probably by a professional scribe; only the address, signature, and postscript are in Smith's handwriting.

2. In 1809 Smith sought to place his vaccine institution on a public statewide basis, and in May he petitioned the Maryland legislature to this end. It voted to authorize a lottery to raise not more than $30,000. Unfortunately this lottery competed with a lottery to raise funds for the Washington Monument which still graces Mt. Vernon Place in Baltimore. Smith's lottery finally took place in 1812, when $12,797.20 were realized. Smith later tried unsuccessfully to establish a national vaccine institution in Washington.   — Bell, "Dr. James Smith," pp. 500–504; Helen C. Brooke, "A Proposal for a Free Vaccine Clinic in Baltimore in 1802," *Bulletin of the History of Medicine* 3 (1935): 83–91.

A-13. Etienne Pariset to — — —, 31 October 1817

Monsieur le comte préfet,

Ma cruelle indisposition m'ôte tout moyen d'éxécuter vos ordres moi même; mais j'ai un bon et zêlé supléant dans Mr. Grignon mon gendre. Mercredi dernier il a fait neuf vaccinations à Arceuil et il a envoyé un enfant en vaccin à Vaugirard chez Mr. Lasfaux, officier de santé, le quel avec cet enfant a du vacciner à Vaugirard et à Issy. Mercredi prochain, une autre vaccination aura lieu à Arceuil. Mr. le maire et Mr. le curé nous secondent de tout leur coeur, en général partout où ce concours de volonté a lieu, les vaccinations ont le plus grand succès. Le même jour, un Enfant de St. Maur sera vacciné à Bicêtre; et son vaccin nous servira pour des vaccinations ultérieures, soit à St. Maur, soit dans les villages environnants. Du reste, les craintes que l'on avait eues à St. Maur ne sont pas fondées. L'éruption qui avait donné l'allarme était celle de la rougeole. Agréez, Monsieur le comte préfet, les sentimens respectueux de votre obeissant serviteur

E Pariset [1]

Bicêtre le 31 8bre 1817

1. Etienne Pariset (1770–1847) was appointed physician at the Hôpital Bicêtre at the time of the Restoration. He became perpetual secretary of the Academy of Medicine in 1822. This letter was transcribed and edited by the late Henry E. Sigerist.

A-14. Sir James Hall to Dr. Alexander J. G. Marcet, 14 Harley St., London, 15 February 1822

Edinburgh Feby. 15. 1822

Dear Sir[1]

On Tuesday we arrived here for the Season[2] and yesterday I received your letter of the 11th recommending Mr. Boissier[3] whom I had the pleasure of meeting last night at the assembly;[4] his conversation revived many circumstances relative to Geneva the memory of which never returns to me without a warm emotion.

Mr. Boissier informed me that your Son had actually had an attack of the Small-pox notwithstanding his previous vaccination by the great Jenner himself. I made it my first business to call on him this morning, and found him so far recovered as to have left his bed-room, with hopes of getting into the open air tomorrow. I had the pleasure to find him in good health and spirits, and seemingly highly delighted with having got so well out of this terrible scrape.[5]

I hope for much satisfaction in this young gentleman's acquaintance during the rest of the Season.

Lady Helen joins me in best compts. to Mrs. Marcet. We hope when you again visit our Northern regions in her company that you will not again forget that Dunglass lies upon the North road.[6]

Yours Sincerely

James Hall[7]

1. See Letter 7, n. 1, for the complete list of the twenty-two letters from Jenner to Marcet published herein.

2. The period when the fashionable world of the eighteenth and early nineteenth centuries assembled for theater, music, and social intercourse.

3. The name of a prominent Geneva family. See J.-A. Galiffe, *Notices généalogiques sur les familles Genevoises* (Geneva, 1829), 1:275–86; 4 (1857): 293–95. I have not been able to ascertain which Boissier was in Edinburgh at this time.

4. Defined as follows in the *OED*: "The public assembly, which formed a regular feature of fashionable life in the 18th century, is described by Chambers (*Cycl.* 1751) as 'a stated and general meeting of the polite persons of both sexes, for the sake of conversation, gallantry, news, and play.'"

5. It is unlikely that Jenner ever learned of this. It is not mentioned in his letter to Marcet

written the following month (see Letter 95). Marcet's son, named François, ultimately became a professor and conseiller d'état in Geneva. — Galiffe, *Notices généalogiques,* 4:313.

6. The main highway between London and Edinburgh.

7. Sir James Hall (1761–1832), geologist and chemist, had been among the first in Britain to accept Lavoisier's new chemical ideas. He had traveled widely and studied on the Continent, including a year in Geneva. He carried out extensive experiments in the attempt to reproduce geological processes. His family seat was at Dunglass in East Lothian, Scotland.

A-15. The Reverend Thomas Pruen to Mr. Walker, Gloucester Journal Office, 31 January 1823

THE LATE DR. JENNER

To the Editor of the Gloucester Journal

Sir

During the greater part of twenty three years uninterrupted friendship, & confidential correspondence with the late eminent character DR. JENNER, he, on a variety of occasions, & with much earnestness, intimated to me his wish, that if it should please God I should survive him, I would, as I knew so much of his life, & sentiments, undertake to be his *Biographer.*[1] The awful event that has just taken place has made me now regard the wish of my departed friend as a *sacred obligation;* the force of which is not lessened by the circumstance, that I was the only one of his very numerous friends who passed the evening of Friday the 24th with him, & had the last conscious pressure of his hand at parting, but a few hours before the unexpected attack from which he never recovered.[2]

I beg leave, therefore, through the medium of your paper, to announce to the friends of Dr. Jenner, & the public, that if I have any remaining strength after the completion of a work ("A VIEW OF THE CHURCH &c") on which I have been labouring for some years past, & part of which has already passed the press, I shall devote whatever time may be spared from my professional duties, to the fulfilment of my much venerated friend's wishes: promised as I am the assistance of his family, & a still free access to the *documents* they possess, few of which are strangers to me.

I venture to hope for the assistance of those, who from their correspondence or intercourse with Dr. Jenner, can furnish any interesting information respecting his habits, or sentiments, & to his medical friends in particular, with many, if not most of whom, I have the honour of a personal acquaintance, I look with a confidence which their liberality in every thing connected with his great discovery — the generous disinterestedness they exhibited thereunto the world, & their to be expected regard for the wishes of our common friend, cannot fail to inspire.

When the great mass of materials that so long a life, & a most extensive correspondence accumulated, has been examined, & arranged, some probable idea may be formed of the *extent*, & necessary *cost* of the publication; but it may be remarked, in advance, that altho such an one will admit of, & it may be presumed in the opinion of most of his friends require, charactaristic [*sic*] embelishments [*sic*], of *Portrait, Views, fac similies* of honourable distinctions, &c&c, yet it will be an object that the copies more immediately devoted to the public shall be at *an usual price;* in order that the private worth of a man, who was as amiable, as he was truly great, may be no less generally known, than his professional merit, & public reputation.

I am Sir   faithfully Yours

Thos Pruen

Rectory Dursley
Jany. 31 1823

Mr. Walker will have the goodness to give this, a *conspicuous place,* in his *Monday's Journal.*[3]

1. For biographical details on Pruen, see Letter 54, n. 1.

2. In the Wellcome Historical Medical Library in London the copy of Thomas Dudley Fosbroke, *Masonic Jennerian Sermon, preached in the Cathedral of Gloucester, August 19, 1823* (Gloucester, 1823) was originally owned by Pruen. At the top of p. 17 near a sentence "they who went to him, as they would to a drama or a lecture, found not an actor or a pedagogue, but a hospitable, kind-hearted, and polished man" are the following comments penned by Pruen: "This was the man with whom *I* had a *close & animated friendship* for near *a quarter of a Century!* I was the *last friend* who partook a *meal* with him on earth! (Jany 24th 1823) I had the last *squeeze of his hand!* Between *us* was the last (generally common) *salutation* 'God bless you!' TP."

3. For unknown reasons, Pruen's letter was never published in the *Gloucester Journal.* Instead the issue published the following Monday, 3 February 1823, contained an anonymous obituary extolling vaccination and Jenner's character which had been written by John Baron, a Gloucester physician whom Jenner had first met in 1808 and who idolized him. The next issue of the *Gloucester Journal* (10 February 1823) contained the following: "Life of the Late Dr. Jenner — We have authority from the Relatives and Trustees of the late Dr. Jenner to state, that in confirmity with his wishes, they have applied to Dr. BARON, of Gloucester, to write the account of the Life, and to arrange for publication the numerous Manuscripts of that distinguished character; and that all the documents in possession of the Family are to be committed to Dr. BARON's care. From that Gentleman, therefore, the public may expect an authentic work, as speedily as his professional avocations will allow him to prepare for the press, the ample and interesting materials with which he is to be furnished, together with those which he himself accumulated during a long and confidential intercourse with Dr. Jenner, and many of his most intimate friends." The result was the two-volume *Life of Edward Jenner, M.D., LL.D., F.R.S., with Illustrations of His Doctrines, and Selections from His Correspondence* by John Baron, M.D., F.R.S. (London, 1827–38).

INDEX

The Index covers all parts of the book, including the footnotes. The note giving the principal identification of a person *follows the name and is italicized.*

Birch, John, *continued*
    Protection, etc. at Ringwood, 127; *The Cowpox Chronicle,* 127; mentioned, xxvii, 27, 28, 58, 70, 71
Blagden, Charles, 6, 7
Blair, William, *43, 128,* 42, 55, 57, 90, 91
    Letter to Okey Belfour, 127
    Letters to, 54, 56
Blane, Sir Gilbert, 121
Blozy, Mr., 130
Blücher, Field Marshal Gebhard Leberecht von, 86
Boerhaave, Hermann, xxi
Boissier, Mr., 134, 135
Bonaparte, Louis (king of Holland), *54,* 53
Bourne, Robert, *92*
Bradley, T., 56, 57
Briggs, Benjamin Church (Milton, Mass.), 131
Briggs, Charles (Milton, Mass.), 131
Briggs, George (Milton, Mass.), 131
Briggs, Joshua (Milton, Mass.), 131
Briggs, Martin (Milton, Mass.), 131
Briggs, Thomas Street (Milton, Mass.), 131
Bristol, smallpox in, 104
Brodie, B. A., 124
Brown, Thomas, *71,* 70
Buckland, William, *89,* 88
Burder, Thomas Harrison, *90*
    Letter to, 90
Burns, Robert, 16

Cabbell, Joseph Carrington (Virginia), 41, 42
Canterbury, Archbishop of, 15
Cardoza, Aaron (Charleston, S.C.), 119
Cardoza, David (Charleston, S.C.), 119
Cardoza, Leah (Charleston, S.C.), 119
Carpue, J. C., 55
Carro, Jean de, *12,* xxii, 19, 21, 77, 78
    Letter to, 9
Cassel, Mr. (murderer), 93
Ceylon, vaccination in, 63
Charleston, South Carolina, vaccination in, 118
Charleston Dispensary, *120,* 118
Cheltenham, *8;* springs, 32, 33–34, 35, 72;

smallpox epidemic, 58; vaccination of poor, 13; mentioned, xxv
Cheltenham Chronicle, 69
"Chevy Chase" (ballad), 18, 19
China, vaccination introduced to, 124, 125
Clinch, Rev. John (Newfoundland), xxi
Cline, Henry, *85,* 84, 127, 128
Cobb, T., 19, 20
    Letters to, 19, 59, 60
Cobb, Mrs. 59
Cockerell, Charles Robert, *68,* 67
Cole, Mary. *See* Berkeley, Lady
Coleridge, Samuel Taylor, 25
College of Physicians (Philadelphia), 43
Colnaghi, Mr.
    Letter to, 76
Colon, Francois, 18
Cooke, 78
Copenhagen, reports on vaccination in, 13, 17, 29, 30
Corvisart, Jean-Nicolas, *130,* xxvi, 67
    Letter to Henri-Marie Husson, 129
Cow, hair from vaccine cow's tail, xxv, xxviii, 83, 84
Cow-Pock Institution (Dublin), 37
Cowpox, description of lesion, 11; relation to smallpox, 11; plate showing pustule, 12; speculation about origin, xxiii, 10, 13, 22
Cross, Mr., 113
Cuming, Miss T., 74
Cuming, Mrs.
    Letter to, 74
Currie, James, *16,* 17, 23
    Letter to, 16
Cushing, Harvey, xxii

Darwin, Charles, 8
Darwin, Erasmus, *Botanic Garden,* 8
Davies, Edward (nephew), 108
Davies, J., 57
Davies, Rev. Robert (nephew), 108
Davies, Rev. Dr. William (nephew), *108,* xxvii, 15, 93, 94, 99
    Letter to, 107
Davies, William (Sr.), *108*
Davies, Dr., 111
Davy, Humphry, xx

Hunter, John, xx, 6, 85; letters to Jenner, xxii
Husson, Henri-Marie, *18,* xxiv, 75, 76, 80, 81, 129, 130
    Letter to, 17
Husson, Captain, *81,* 75, 76, 80
Hydatids, speculation about, xxv, 79, 96
Hyde, Mrs., 82

India, vaccination in, 19
Ingram, William (Berkeley gamekeeper), 94
Inoculation. *See* Variolation
Institute of the History of Medicine, Johns Hopkins, xxii

Jacobs, Henry Barton, *xxii;* collection of Jennerian books and letters, xix-xx, 28, 84
Jacobs Collection, William H. Welch Medical Library, 28, 84
Jeanroy, 130
Jefferson, Thomas, 74
Jenner, Anne (sister), 108
Jenner, Catherine (daughter), 7, 8, 65, 66, 68, 89, 93, 96, 99, 104
Jenner, Edward (For full chronological data, consult the Contents where a summary of each letter is given), letters also briefly summarized, xxii-xxvi; apology for delinquent correspondence, 7, 13, 21, 28, 57, 74-75; bust by Manning, 26; portrait by Northcote, 79; "Temple of Vaccinia" at Berkeley, 80; depicted as a monster, 38; M.D. from St. Andrews, 39; inscribed copy of Ring's *Answer to Dr. Moseley* in Welch Medical Library, 28
    Domestic Concerns: financial disappointment, 20; residence in Cheltenham, 21; godfather, 70, 71, 94, 95; advice to son Robert about wine, 91-92, 93; son Edward's illness and death, 47, 48, 58, 59, 61, 64, 66, 67; concern about son Robert's health, 79-80, 83, 86, 91
    Medical Practice and Theories: arranges to vaccinate a child, 41; vaccinated the poor at Cheltenham, 13; vaccinated Marcet's son, 134; proposes that smallpox inocula-

tion be banned, 63; instructions about vaccination, 36, 114; pays publishing expenses of vaccination supporters, 27, 62, 64, 65; medical prescriptions, 20, 59-60; advice to female vaccinator, 23; consultant, 59, 60-61, 72, 74, 113-114; medical attendant of Lord Berkeley, 73; comment on eyes, 7-8; interest in liver inflammation, 78; performed animal dissections, 79; curious about lymphatics, 90; speculations about mother's milk, 94; hydatids, 96, 97; theory that the stomach governs the body, 7, 8, 96
    Medical Writings: paper to Fleece Medical Society on acute rheumatism leading to heart disease, 24, 25; *Inquiry into the Causes and Effects of the Variolae Vaccinae,* 3, 8, 9, 10, 12, 15, 22, 80, 83, 84; *Further Observations on the Variolae Vaccinae,* 10, 12; *Instructions for Vaccine Inoculation,* 16, 17, 118, 120; *On the Varieties and Modifications of the Vaccine Pustule,* 22; *Letter . . . on the Influence of Artificial Eruptions,* 105, 106, 107, 111, 113; publications on the effect of herpetic eruptions on the vaccine pustule, 36, 37; letter to Robert Willan, 32, 33; preparing an anonymous publication, 26; proposes republishing vaccination articles in *Medical and Physical Journal,* 29; papers in C. H. Parry's possession, 24; paper on smallpox of foetus, 45, 46, 49, 52, 53; circular letter, 103, 104, 110, 111; notebook, 46; letter reprinted in *Charleston Times,* 119
    Non-medical Activities: balloon flight, xxv, 3; experiments with blood as manure, 4-6; report on mating of dog and fox, 4; paper on bird migration, 6, 7; cuckoo observations published in *Philosophical Transactions,* 6, 7; paper on dog distemper, 45, 46, 49, 52, 53; functioning as magistrate in Berkeley, xxv, 75, 92, 93, 94, 111; House of Commons witness *re* Berkeley succession, 73; exchange of war prisoners, 66, 67, 75, 80-81; introductory letters for British travelers, 41, 67, 68; geological interests, 62, 89, 96, 98, 101, 107; horticultural interests, 66, 83, 89, 112

St. Andrews University, M.D. diplomas, 38, 39
Saunders, William, *48,* 47, 51, 58, 61, 62, 65, 87, 108, 110
Savage, John, *42,* 41
Schmidtmeyer, Mrs., 41
Seager, Mr., 69
Shakespeare, William, 7, 83
Sheppard, Miss, 93
Shoolbred, John, 41, 42
Shorter, 59
Shrapnell, Henry, *90,* 89
Shrapnell, William F., *7,* 6
Shriver, David (Jr.) (Westminster, Md.), 132
    James Smith letter to, 132
Sigerist, Henry E., editor, *Letters of Jean de Carro to Alexandre Marcet,* xxii, 130, 134
Smith, James, *133,* xxvi
    Letter to David Shriver, Jr., 132
Smith, John (Milton, Mass.), 131
Smith, Mr. (Charleston, S.C.), 117
Smallpox, extermination of, xxiv, 20, 24, 123; eradicated by World Health Organization, xix; related to cowpox, 11; inoculation (*See* Variolation)
Smallpox and Inoculation Hospital (London), contamination of cowpox vaccine, 10–11, 12, 63
Spain, royal expedition to bring vaccination to New World, 31, 32, 33
Squirrel, Robert, *28,* 27, 29, 31, 33
Stanger, Christopher, *123,* 122
Stanhope, Mr., 75
Staunton, Sir George Leonard, 124
Staunton, Sir George Thomas, *124,* xxvii
    Letter by, 124
Stevenson, Lloyd G., 82
Stibbs (Cheltenham), 68
Stuart, John Ferdinand Smyth, *38; Letter to Lord Henry Petty,* 38
Swann, John, *33,* 32, 35

Taylor, David, 15, 16
Taylor, James, 70, 71
Temkin, Owsei, 60
"Temple of Vaccinia," 80
Thackeray, Frederic, *48,* 47, 50

Thompson (Cheltenham), 35
Thomson, John (Halifax), *64; Cheap Tract on the Cow-Pox,* 63, 64; mentioned, xxiv
    Letter to, 63
Thouret, 130
Tilloch, Alexander, *76*
Typhus, remedy for, 16, 17

Vaccination, in America, 99; Bengal, 42; Ceylon, 63; Charleston, South Carolina, 118; China, xxvii, 124, 125; Copenhagen, 13, 17, 29, 30; Dublin, 37; France, xxvi, 18, 129, 130, 133; Geneva, 30; Holland, 53; India, 19, 49; Italy, 48; Latin America, 31, 32, 33; Liverpool, 16; Lyons, 30, 31; Madras, 43; Mediterranean, 18; Milton, Massachusetts, 131; Sweden, 53; Vienna, 10; arm-to-arm, 41; number of British vaccinations in 1799, 11; performed by laymen, including women, xxiii, 22, 38, 114; word coined by Richard Dunning, 79; early use of word, 119; skin eruption following, 13; experiment at London Foundling Hospital, 122; lottery in Baltimore, 132–133; anti-vaccinists (*See* under names): John Birch, J. Davies, George Lipscomb, Benjamin Moseley, William Rowley, Robert Squirrel, John Ferdinand Smyth Stuart
Vaccine inoculation. *See* Vaccination
Vaccine Pock Institution (London), 25
Vaccine virus, preparation of, 10; time to collect, 13; preservation, 42; method of transporting, 128; ready to cross Atlantic, 99; speculation about origin, 11, 14, 22
Vaccinia virus. *See* Vaccine virus
Variolation, responsible for smallpox epidemics, 63; mentioned, 32, 34, 51, 117
Viborg, E., 14
Vienna, vaccination in, 10
Vigel, J., 93

Wait, Miss, 71
Wake, Mrs., 45–46
Walker, John, *33,* 18, 32, 43, 44
Walker, Richard, 95, 96
Walker (*Gloucester Journal*), 135, 136
Wall, Martin, *92,* 91

Ward, John
  Letters to, 97, 102
Warner, Mr. (Charleston, S.C.), 117
Washbourn, Rev. Dr., 3
Waterhouse, Benjamin, 118, 119, 120
Wathen, Samuel, 14, 15
Watts, Mrs., 31
Webb, Miss, 102
Weir, 66
Wellcome Historical Medical Library (London), 42, 50, 69, 80, 86, 136
White, Joshua Elder, *119*
  David Ramsay letter to, 118

Wilberforce, William, *55,* 70
Willan, Robert, *39,* 16, 29, 32, 33, 38, 43
Willemoes, Frederick Wilhelm, *30,* 29, 31
William H. Welch Medical Library (Baltimore, Md.), given Jenner letters, xix, xxii
Winsloew, Frederik Christian, *17*
Woodville, William, *12,* 25
Worthington, Rev. Dr. Richard, *84,* 15
  Letters to, 82, 98
Worthington, Miss, 83, 102
Wyndham, Sir George O'Brien, 48

Yelloly, John, 33